Negative Calorie
Lose 20 Pounds in 30 Days

©Ala Silva

Forward

I would like to thank you for purchasing the book "Negative Calorie."

In this book you will find proven strategies to help you lose weight in an efficient and sustainable way. Eating all natural, organic and nutrient dense foods that have high quality calories is the key to finding balance in your life and shedding the extra pounds once and for all.

We are going to start by first laying the foundation of the "Negative Calorie Diet" through delving deeper into the different types of calories, the proven negative calorie foods and their benefits.

The second part contains simple, healthy and mouthwatering recipes made using negative calorie ingredients that will turbo charge your weight loss efforts.

As you go through this eBook feel free to take notes as you go along as this is the diet that changes your life from now henceforth!

Table of Contents

Lunch Recipes..107

Introduction

Is it for vanity or are we genuinely concerned about our health? This is the primary question when it comes to wanting to lose weight. In America alone, there are over 400 diets and counting that promise to give you the body you have been dreaming of; and this begs the question - why **are we still so fat?**

The truth is, most diets on the market are not sustainable as they are based on deprivation – YOU CANT EAT THIS AMOUNT OF FOOD BECAUSE ITS GOING TO MAKE YOU FAT... and quite frankly the weight loss foods on most diets are bland and simply boring, explaining why most people jump ship even before hitting the half-way milestone in their diet.

You have probably been on at least one diet and the fact that you are reading the "Negative Calorie Diet" means it didn't quite work as you had hoped for. Now, the question is, what makes the "Negative Calorie Diet" stand out from other diets?

First, the negative diet is not the conventional diet, in the sense that it's not time based; it's not restrictive in terms of the number of calories you can take in a day and it doesn't impose unrealistic demands on you. This diet is in every sense a way of life. Once you are on it, you will never want to turn back!

What is the negative calorie diet?

This is an eating plan that is built on a 30 day plan aimed at jumpstarting healthy lifestyle changes for the long run. It first starts by cleansing your body of all toxins that are weighing it down in readiness for the immense benefits of a nutrient-dense, organic and whole foods diet.

This is followed by delicious recipes that are built on protein and supplemented by organic negative calorie foods, super foods and spices bursting with flavor, fat-burning and health promoting results.

Negative calorie foods will help shred extra fat, they will boost your metabolism – rate at which your body burns calories and they will help you stay full after eating them – meaning you're going to eat less food.

With the "Negative Calorie Diet" we can finally say that we have solved the mystery of weight loss!

Chapter 1:

Food Psychology

From this point forward, you're going to exercise the first principle of the Negative Calorie Diet – before anything goes into your mouth, ask yourself, and "is this a negative calorie food?"

If you answered yes, then you know you are on the right track as the food in question is going to provide your body with high quality nutrition to stay healthy and supply you with the energy to go about your daily activities. And the best part, you can eat as much as you need to get full. You are now in a 'no-calorie counting zone!'

If on the other hand you answered no, then you want to stay as far away from that food as possible because it's not going to provide even an ounce of nourishment to your body and further along the way you may develop chronic illnesses and you are definitely not going to lose weight!

Not all calories are created equal

Many of us are familiar with the basic science of weight loss – for you to lose weight, you've got to use more calories than what you are eating. A traditional negative balance, which most of us are familiar with, is achieved by reducing your caloric intake so your body is forced to tap into the stored fat in your body for energy. Unfortunately, this approach requires serious food restrictions that are hunger inducing and not forgetting the wearisome calorie counting.

But, what if there is a better way to create a negative calorie balance in your body without having to cut or count calories but eat as much as is necessary to make you full?

Well, we're in luck because it just so happens there is!

And all you have to do is eat organic, nutrient-dense, real and wholesome foods.

Eating high quality calories from natural and wholesome calories fuels your body and in turn helps you burn fat. On the other hand, eating low quality calories from processed and starchy foods slows down your metabolism and leads to weight gain and a host of chronic illnesses

The 'calorie myth' is one of the most persistent... and perhaps the most damaging. It' the idea that calories make the most important part of any diet and that where those calories came from doesn't really matter. This goes further to say that it doesn't matter if you eat 100calories of broccoli or ice cream, the two will have the same effect on your weight.

But when we look at how your body operates, it's not that simple. The truth is, different foods are handled by your body differently and most importantly different macronutrients have a major effect on your hormones and brain centers that control your hunger and general eating behavior.

What you eat has a huge impact on your body's biological processes that are in charge of what and how much you eat. The bottom line is, different sources of calories can have very different effects on energy expenditure, hormones, hunger and the brain regions governing food intake.

While calories are important, you don't need to count them or be constantly aware of them in order to lose weight. Simple changes in the food you eat by adopting negative calorie foods will yield you better results compared to calorie restriction. This is a concept we are going to expound on all through the book.

Whole foods factor

The negative calorie foods are essentially whole foods – foods that have not been altered from their natural state through processing or those that have been minimally altered to make them edible.

What's essential to understand is that calories from whole foods are high quality calories. In the same light, processed foods that have been significantly changed from their natural states contain low quality calories.

The best part about eating whole foods is that their calories are not stored as fat in your body unlike calories from processed foods. You can enjoy eating large portions of whole foods and continue losing weight!

The metabolism factor

Metabolism is your body's engine. During the day your body activates catabolic metabolism – providing energy for all your waking hours' activities and the functioning of all your body's components.

At night, it activates anabolic metabolism – providing energy to repair and replace the billions of worn out cells as well as any damaged or stressed tissues. All these happen when you are sleeping.

Metabolism regulates how your body uses calories and this depends on your calorie needs, the availability of calories and the quality of calories.

There are several ways of revving up your metabolism. Weight or strength training boosts your metabolism by building muscle which is a fat burning tissue. Detoxifying your body is another way to boost your metabolism as it cleanses your liver which is your body's main fat-burning organ, allowing it to work optimally.

Digestion is another important factor in determining your rate of metabolism. By eating whole foods you enable your digestive system to absorb all the nutrition from your food and thus provide your body with high quality fuel.

Thermogenic foods also play a vital role in metabolism as well as digestion. Thermogenesis is simply the process by which your body generates heat as you digest food. Did you know that you can burn up to 800 calories through thermogenesis? This is according to the Mayo Clinic.

Cruciferous veggies such as broccoli and cauliflower as well as high protein foods are thermogenic. By eating them, you instantly create a negative calorie balance in your body.

The full factor – satiating your hunger

Who needs a gastric by-pass when we have negative calorie foods? These foods are satiating, making you feel full faster and so you eat less of them. What makes negative calorie foods satiating is the fact that they have a very high fiber and water content (fruits and veggies) and some are also high in protein (lean meats).

If you have been on any diet before, you can attest to feeling like someone purposely sent hunger to make your diet fail. Unfortunately when we reach these crazy levels of hunger the first foods we seek out are fast digesting high calorie diets. This is an evolutionary trait that is wired in our systems to help out when we feel like we are starving. This explains why when on a diet and feel ravenously hungry the first thing you want to do is bury your face in a creamy donut.

18

Processed foods such as refined carbs, white rice, breakfast cereals are primarily made up of starch molecules which are immediately converted into sugar by your body. This fast digestion causes a spike in blood sugar which is followed by a fast and hard hitting crash.

In contrast negative calorie foods provide you with a slow and steady source of fuel, keeping you energized all through the day. No more sugar high and sugar low rollercoasters or binge moments with negative calorie foods.

In summary, negative calorie foods are endowed with high quality calories that fill you up and rev up your metabolism. The result? Quick and sustainable weight loss with not an ounce of deprivation.

Metabolic secrets – the eat all you want benefit of the "Negative Calorie Diet"

So far we have seen that negative calorie foods naturally put your body on a negative calorie balance without having to count or obsess over calories. You can eat to your fill but always ensure you have at least one of the negative calorie foods in every meal. (We're going to look at these foods in the next chapter)

Aside from heaping on negative calorie foods you can rev up your fat burning machine by adding healthy and lean proteins to your meals. Proteins take longer to digest compared to carbs and fats and thus require more energy to do that.

Look at it in this sense: if you eat a 500 calorie meal that has a healthy serving of protein like chicken, fish or meat you can expect to use up 125 calories through digestion alone. Additionally, you get the essential amino acids that help your body repair and grow muscle.

Spicing your food naturally is another amazing way to boost your metabolism. We are going to look at some of the fat-burning spices you can incorporate into your cooking in the next chapter.

Here is the super metabolic boosting formula from eating only:

Negative Calorie Foods + Healthy Protein + Natural Spices = A Tasty Way To Lose Weight!

Chapter 2:

Cleansing and Detoxifying Au Naturel

Feeling out of sync or sluggish? Are you in constant battle with fatigue, skin breakouts, aches, unexplainable pains and digestive problems and not forgetting, a constant struggle with weight loss? Well, your body is placing a distress call and it's about time for a great detox.

This is the first thing you should do before embarking on the Negative Calorie Diet. For faster health and weight loss results, you should first cleanse your system.

As with all the principles of the Negative Calorie Diet, we are going to do the detox au natural. By removing and eliminating all toxins from your body and feeding on a fresh, natural and wholesome diet, you will not only protect your body from disease but you will also renew your ability to attain optimum health and set yourself up for successful and sustainable weight loss.

Cleansing and detoxifying naturally

Basically, cleansing and detoxifications means cleaning your blood. This is achieved by removing impurities and free radicals from the blood in your liver, where toxins are usually processed for elimination. Your body also eliminates toxins through your intestines, kidneys, lymphs, lungs and skin.

However, when your body is compromised, impurities are not filtered in the right way and every cell in your body is adversely affected.

A healthy detox program helps your body's natural cleansing process by:

- Stimulating your liver to eliminate toxins from your body
- Resting your organs through periodic fasting
- Improving your blood circulation
- Promoting elimination of toxins through your kidneys, intestines and skin; and
- Rejuvenating your body with healthy negative calorie foods

The reason natural detoxification works is because it addresses the specific needs of individual cells which are the smallest units of human life.

How do you know that your body needs detoxification?

Today, with more toxins in our environment than ever before, it's essential to detox in order to keep our bodies functioning smoothly. We recommend that you detox your body at least once a year. You know that you need to detox if you experience symptoms such as:

- Allergies
- Unexplained fatigue
- Regular bloating
- Menstrual irregularities
- Sluggish elimination
- Mental confusion such as memory lapses
- Irritated skin
- Puffy eyes

How to detox

The first step is to lighten your toxic load by eliminating all processed foods (refined and artificial and sugars, refined and bleached flours, hydrogenated and trans fats, gluten, chemicals in food and genetically modified foods), cigarettes, alcohol and coffee, all of which are received as toxins by your body and are an obstacle to the normal functioning of your body.

You should also minimize or better yet, eliminate the use of chemical-based detergents, household products, deodorant, and skin care products; and substitute them with organic and all natural alternatives.

Stress is another deterrent to good health as it triggers the release of stress hormones in your system. In large amounts these stress hormones override your detoxification enzymes in your liver. Meditation and yoga are some of the methods to help you deal with stress the right way.

The best ways to help your body detoxify

1. Drink at least eight glasses of water a day.
2. Eat plenty of negative calorie foods that are high fiber and that are organically grown. Radish, beets and edible seaweed are detoxifying super foods.
3. Take vitamin C rich foods. Vitamin C helps your body produce glutathione, a liver compound that eliminates toxins.
4. Cleanse and protect your liver by taking herbs such as milk thistle, dandelion root and burdock
5. Practice swimmers breathing (deep breathing) to allow oxygen to circulate more effectively and completely through your system.

6. Go to a sauna to allow your body to eliminate toxins through perspiration
7. Occasionally practice hydrotherapy by taking an extremely hot shower (as hot as you can handle) for five minutes; allowing the water to run down your body, especially your back. Follow this with very cold water for 30 seconds. Repeat this 3 times then take a nap for 30 minutes.
8. Dry brush your skin to drive toxins through your pores – look for special brushes in natural products department stores.
9. Exercising is a great way to detoxify. Fast jump roping and yoga are very effective. 30 minutes every day is enough time for an effective workout.

Try out this cleansing tea to help your body in driving out toxins. Combine this detox tea with the negative calorie recipes we are going to be looking at in Chapter 4.

All day fat flushing tea

- Combine 8 cups of brewed green tea (unsweetened) with slices of lime, lemon and orange in a large pitcher.
- Serve over ice or take it hot. You can refrigerate for up to 3 days.
- Take 1 pitcher of this fat flushing tea a day for 5 days.

Give natural cleansing and detoxification an honest try and you are going to love how the Negative Calorie Diet is going to work for you in your weight loss journey and also in helping you transition to healthier long term eating habits.

Chapter 3:

The Negative Calorie Foods Unmasked!

Nature has gifted us with tons and tons of healthy and nutrient-rich foods. But unfortunately, many of us have been avoiding natural foods and have instead been eating foods out of boxes that come with an expiry label.

Not to worry, the Negative Calorie Diet is here to help you become one with nature and for this purpose, we are going to look at 10 of the most potent negative calorie foods. This is not to say that they are the only healthy foods, but they are the ones that will help you meet your weight loss goals faster.

So, how did we come up with these 10 super foods?

Nutritional profile

These negative calorie foods are endowed with nutrients such as vitamins, fiber, protein and essential minerals that will rev up your metabolism and also promote a healthy lifestyle.

- **Research**

Each of the 10 foods has been proven to be thermogenic, satiating and to promote health.

- **Multipurpose**

You can easily source these 10 negative calorie foods and the best part is that you can use them either for breakfast, lunch or dinner. You can also eat most of them without cooking, making them perfect even for those days you don't feel like cooking.

The moment of truth! Here are the 10 negative calorie foods that we've been talking about.

1. Almonds

These are little powerhouses of nutrition and one of the keys to losing weight once and for all. A handful of almonds (approximately 10 almonds) is only 78 calories. Additionally, they are endowed with fiber, monounsatured fats (good fats) vitamins and zinc which helps curb sugar cravings.

Here are effective ways of including almonds in the Negative Calorie Diet:

- Substitute your regular snack for a handful of almonds
- Eat a few almonds before dinner to reduce your appetite owing to their high fiber content
- Add almonds to your breakfast muesli or porridge for a healthy and fiber rich breakfast that will keep you full all through the morning.

2. Apples

Apples have immense nutritional benefits that they justify the "an apple a day..." adage. These amazing fruits keep hunger at bay using very few calories. Additionally, they are endowed with pectin – a type of fiber and antioxidants that get rid of free radicals. They are also a good source of Vitamin C which helps boost your immunity.

Apples have also been shown to protect against and reduce symptoms of cardiovascular diseases and metabolic syndrome. You can also use an apple as an exercise extender by eating it before your workout for increased endurance.

Keep the skin on to retain the full amount of fiber which can be as much as 5g.

3. Berries

Blueberries, raspberries, blackberries, strawberries and cherries are packed full of nutrients and are very low in sugar compared to most fruit, which is the reason why they are lauded as some of the greatest fat-burners.

The fiber in berries helps a great deal with satiety and their high antioxidant power helps eliminate toxins, free radicles and stop premature aging. With all the vitamins, nutrients and minerals berries provide, they are a great negative calorie diet to incorporate into your diet.

4. Celery

Roughly 75 percent of celery is water and the remaining 25 percent is comprised of fiber. Celery therefore provides you with fewer calories than what your body will burn as it digests it. It is also an excellent source of fiber that does a great job keeping you fuller for longer and reducing the urge to snack on non-negative calorie foods.

Aside from weight loss, the other health benefit of celery is that it's endowed with natural nutrients such as Vitamins

A, C and K. It also has antioxidant properties that improve your heart's health.

Furthermore, celery's high fiber content improves your digestive tract's health.

5. Cucumbers

Like many of the negative calorie foods, cucumber is mostly made up of water helping you burn fat faster. Additionally, you can take cucumber right before your workout to stay energized and hydrated.

You can also munch on cucumber slices on a hot summer afternoon when dipped in a healthy nut hummus.

Cucumbers have also been shown to reduce inflammation in the body as they are naturally endowed with anti-inflammatory enzymes that act in the same way as anti-inflammatory drugs like ibuprofen.

It is also a good source of Vitamin C which improves your body's ability to resist bacterial and virus infection.

6. Cruciferous veggies

Cruciferous veggies such as broccoli, lettuce and cauliflower are some of the best foods you can eat as they only contain 30 calories per serving. They also have a very high fiber content that helps keep you full longer.

Broccoli for instance has a high protein content, equal to that found in rice but with only a fraction of the calories found in rice.

If you are looking to boost your immunity and your body's ability to fight off infections, then cruciferous veggies are a great negative calorie addition to your lifestyle.

Broccoli is also an amazing source of selenium, zinc and beta-carotene which not only strengthen your immunity but also improve your body's overall function.

The trick with cruciferous veggies is to cook them for as little time as possible or better still eat them raw in a salad for you to get the maximum nutritional benefits.

7. Citrus fruits

Citrus fruits are essentially water with healthy nutrients and roughage thrown in. citrus fruits have 60 percent water content with the rest being healthy fiber that boosts digestion. Grapefruit in particular is endowed with pectin, a special type of fiber, which not only fills you up but also reduces arterial hardening thus promoting heart health.

Vitamin C and phytonutrients such as limonoids are another great reason to have consume citrus fruits on a regular basis.

8. Watermelon

This is the most popular fruit on a hot summer afternoon due to its high water content. Watermelon is extremely low in calories and does a great job in helping with weight loss. One of the reasons that make this fruit an amazing fat burner is that it is an extremely rich source of B vitamins which boost your energy levels thus reducing your desire to eat extra foods – which you may be tempted to do when you are feeling tired and sluggish.

Watermelon has a high fiber and protein content and thus has the ability to rev up your metabolism compared to most fruits.

Additionally, it is a great source of lycopene – an antioxidant that protects your body against cancers of the breast, respiratory system, colon and womb.

Don't wait too long, go get yourself a crunchy and juicy bite!

9. Chili peppers

Chili peppers are endowed with capsaicin, a compound which boosts your metabolism thus causing you to burn fat faster for a while even after consumption. Chili peppers have very few calories and so they help you burn more calories than what they contain.

Most people also tend to feel less hungry after consuming meals cooked with hot chili peppers making them a great choice when you are looking to reduce your appetite.

Habanero peppers are especially very rich in capsaicin and you should therefore have more of these.

10. Asparagus

Grilled asparagus is so tasty you can even forget you are eating a vegetable. Now, asparagus is a great detoxifier owing to the fact that it contains diuretic properties that help drive toxins from your body. Eating asparagus also revs up your metabolism as it is one of the super negative calorie foods.

Asparagus is an essential addition to a pregnant woman's diet as it is a very rich source of folate which helps reduce the risk of birth defects such as spina bifida.

It also helps reduce bloating and tummy discomforts thereby aiding in digestion. Asparagus is a true super food!

Here are other fat-blasting negative calorie foods that should also feature in your diet.

- **Cabbage**

This veggie is an amazing source of fiber and vitamin C. enjoy both the green and red varieties as a wrap, in a smoothie, salad or soup.

- **Carrots**

Carrots come in different colors – red, white, purple and yellow. They are renowned for their high beta-carotene content. Use them as a potato substitute by making carrot fries or use them in a roll, a stew or better yet, eat them raw.

- **Bananas**

In addition to their high potassium content, bananas are also a very good source of fiber with about 3 grams. Half a banana is a great addition to a balanced breakfast meal.

- **Black beans**

A cup of black beans have a whopping 30 grams of fiber! It is a very versatile ingredient that can be used in a variety of recipes such as casseroles, salads, stews and brownies.

- **Lentils**

This is an extremely nutritious legume with a cup having 16 grams of fiber. You can make a lentil burger or use it to make a spicy lentil bowl for a nutritious and filling dinner.

- **Oatmeal**

This wholegrain is an amazing source of fiber, folate among other nutrients. Make oatmeal porridge, pancakes or muffins.

- **Peas**

Aside from being a rich source of protein, they are also a great fiber option with a cup containing up to 11 grams. You can make a spicy snack, as part of a stew or as a risotto topping.

- **Pineapple**

A medium sized pineapple can have up to 13 grams of fiber, making it an ideal juicy and cooling fruit option on a hot day. You can use it to make a smoothie, eat it as is or to make infused water.

- **Spinach**

Packed with fiber and nutrients, spinach is a great leafy green to include in your diet. You can use it in smoothies, stir-fries or to make healthy brownies.

- **Sweet potatoes**

These tubers are rich in vitamins and they can have up to 4 grams of fiber in one small-medium sized tuber. Boil it, add it to your casserole, tacos or broth.

Spice up your food with these negative calorie natural spices

- **Black pepper**

It aids with sluggish digestion and it helps other foods to get absorbed into the bloodstream faster.

- **Cayenne pepper**

This is a medicinal spice that has been used for thousands of years and it boosts your fat burning rate by up to 25percent.

- **Cardamom**

This is a natural detoxifier, immunity booster and digestive aid.

- **Cinnamon**

It helps lessen insulin production so your body doesn't convert sugar into fat and it is also a great appetite suppressant and anti-fungal to help treat infections faster.

- **Ginger**

It revs up your metabolism and settles nausea and indigestion

- **Garlic**

It helps lower your blood pressure and also breaks up fat molecules thus reducing bad cholesterol level in your body. It is also a good metabolism booster.

- **Turmeric**

This is a medicinal spice that has been used for centuries. It fights inflammation, and cancer cells and also helps normalize blood sugar levels. It also boost your metabolic rate thus helping you burn fat faster.

- **Mustard**

It fills you up thus reducing appetite and also increases your metabolic rate.

- **Horseradish**

This is a metabolism booster and an effective fat burner.

The ultimate negative calorie food!

Water

Water has zero calories and it can help control your appetite in addition to fueling thermogenesis. Taking two large glasses of water can increase your metabolic rate by up to 30 percent in just 10 minutes; this is according to research done at Humboldt State University in Arcata, California.

Also taking water before meals helps you lower weight faster as it means you are not going to eat as much as you would have had you not taken the water.

Often times, thirst can be mistaken for hunger pangs so next time you feel hungry in the middle of the afternoon, swig a glass of water and it might just do the trick.

Water also helps the detoxification process by helping in driving out the toxins. Additionally, the oxygen component of water offers your brain and entire body some energy boost.

For faster weight loss, take a minimum of 8 glasses of water every day and ensure you take a glass before every meal in order to suppress your appetite.

There you have it! Negative calorie foods to kick start your weight loss and healthy living journey.

Let us now jump into the recipe section for mouthwatering and super simple recipes that will be ready within no time. Get your apron ready!

Chapter 4:
1 FULL Month Meal Plan

You've heard it said; 'failure to plan is planning to fail.' Whether you are only cooking for one or for your entire family, taking the time to sit and plan for what you are going to eat for the coming week will not just save you time, money and effort; it will also enhance your healthy eating habits.

Four reasons why you should have a meal plan:

- You will culture healthy eating habits

The main premise of The Anti-Inflammatory Diet is to eat food that is going to help your body fight off destructive inflammation and also protect you from chronic inflammation. When you have a carefully set out meal plan, you won't need to resort to ordering takeout as you will have healthy food waiting for you at home.

Habit is second to nature and as you get used to planning healthy meals, you will soon forget about the processed and inflammatory foods that used to slow you down.

- You become an informed shopper

The specific ingredients listed in the recipes you are going to make will teach you the healthiest ingredients that you need to buy. Forget about overly processed food that has got no nutritional value, you focus will now shift to fresh, natural, nutrient dense foods.

- You will save time and money

When you know exactly what you are going to cook, you will shop for ingredients more efficiently and thus save more money. You won't also have to waste time brainstorming on what to cook as it's already planned.

- You will eat a variety of food

Planning your meals will allow you to eat something new almost every day, if not every day, instead of eating one thing all week. If you have a family, they are sure to dig this method and it will give them something to look forward to every day.

One Month Meal Plan

Meal Plan – Week One		
	Monday	**Tuesday**	**Wednesday**
Breakfast	Berry breakfast bowl	Blueberry quinoa power breakfast muffins	Energizing Acai Bowl
Lunch	Zesty Chicken Bites	A veggie extravaganza!	Green Bean Salad with Walnuts
Dinner	Herbed chicken and veggie stir-fry	Citrusy baked salmon with bulgur and asparagus	Wild Grilled Salmon
Thursday	**Friday**	**Saturday**	**Sunday**
Smoked salmon-egg white sandwich	Cherry-nut oatmeal	Healthy herbed frittata	Breakfast Fruit Salad
Avocado Egg Salad	Chipotle Chicken Stuffed Sweet Potatoes	Squash Salad	Mexican Romaine Salad
Mexican Beef Stuffed Peppers	Greek Roast Lamb	Curried Vegetables with Cauliflower 'Rice'	Baked Beef with Mushroom and Squash

	Monday	**Tuesday**	**Wednesday**
Breakfast	Apple & Sweet Potato Pancakes	Sweet Potato & Bacon Stir Fry	Breakfast Sausage and Mushroom Casserole
Lunch	Mediterranean Grilled Vegetables	Turkish Salad with Pomegranate Molasses	Green Mango Salad
Dinner	Tuna Burgers	Spicy Beef Roast	Wholesome Pizza
Thursday	**Friday**	**Saturday**	**Sunday**
Yummy Steak Muffins	Coconut Muffins	White and Green Quiche	Deviled Eggs
Apple Spinach Salad	Roasted Carrots with Curried Cashew Sauce	Spicy Italian Salad	Tuna - Watercress Salad
Asian Style Curry	Thai Red Curry	Southwestern Meatloaf	Lemon Zested Shrimps

Meal Plan – Week Two

Meal Plan – Week Three			
	Monday	**Tuesday**	**Wednesday**
Breakfast	Delicious Spicy Pumpkin Patties	Apple & Cinnamon Porridge	Baked Eggs
Lunch	Baked Sweet Potato Fries	Crunchy Kale Salad with Avocado Dressing	Roasted Artichoke Hearts with Lemon and Olives
Dinner	Chicken Veggie Soup	Sweet & Sour Pork	Crispy Duck & Baked Vegetables
Thursday	**Friday**	**Saturday**	**Sunday**
Yummy Zucchini Latkes	Turkey Breakfast Scramble	Pork and Egg Breakfast Casserole	Zucchini and Steak Casserole
Chard Skillet with Eggs	Moroccan-Style Grilled Ground Beef	Apple-Walnut Chicken Salad	Charmila (North African–Style Tomato Poached Eggs)
Roasted Rack of Lamb with Blackberry Sauce	Lamb Ragu with Celery Root Pasta	Pork Meatloaf with Sun Dried Tomato & Mushrooms	Caribbean Salad with Monk Fish

	Monday	Tuesday	Wednesday
Meal Plan – Week Four			
Breakfast	Beef Breakfast Casserole	"Toast" Negative Calorie Style	Breakfast Bowl
Lunch	Moroccan Fish Tagine	Stuffed Acorn Squash with Sage and Thyme	Grilled Salmon with Citrus Marinade
Dinner	Chili Bison Stew	Fried Pork on Turnip Rice	Island Salmon with Mange Chili Salsa
Thursday	**Friday**	**Saturday**	**Sunday**
Chocolate Banana Bowl	Ham and Veggie Frittata Muffins	Tomato and Avocado Omelet	Spicy Sausage Wrapped Eggs
Bacon and Vegetable Frittata	Super Tender Stewed Chicken with Vegetables	Chilean Chacero Salad	Classic Roast Chicken
Pumpkin & Sun-dried Tomato Pork Stew	Beef and Broccoli Stir Fry	Cilantro Lime Halibut	Slow Cooker Chicken Chili Verde

Chapter 4: Recipes

Smoothie recipes

Fountain of youth smoothies

Ingredients

1 cup roughly chopped kale, with the stems discarded

1 kiwi fruit, peeled

1 frozen banana

1/8 honey dew melon, chopped

1 cup baby spinach

1 avocado, chopped

½ cup unsweetened natural almond milk, chilled

Directions

1. Combine all the ingredients in your blender and pulse until desired consistency is achieved.
2. Serve in a tall glass.
3. Enjoy!

Fiberrific Berry Oat smoothie

Ingredients

½ cup frozen blueberries

4 large, ripe strawberries, hulled

110 ml unsweetened natural cranberry juice

150ml non-fat, unsweetened vanilla Greek yogurt

1 tbsp. oat bran

1 tbsp. freshly squeezed lime juice

Natural honey or pure maple syrup to taste (optional)

Directions

1. Mix all the ingredients in your blender and pulse until you get a smooth puree-like consistency.
2. Enjoy!

A Hint of Mint Kefir Smoothie

Ingredients

2 cups unsweetened organic kefir

1 cup freshly chopped cucumber

¼ cup fresh mint leaves

½ tsp ground cumin

2-3 tbsp. freshly squeezed lime juice

A pinch of fine sea salt

Cumin seeds for topping

Directions

1. Combine all the ingredients together in your blender and pulse until smooth.
2. Serve immediately.
3. Enjoy!

Note: This smoothie is a great detoxifier and a healthy source of calcium and protein.

Belly Fat Loss Smoothie

Ingredients

½ avocado

½ cup frozen blueberries

½ frozen banana

¼ tsp cinnamon

1 tbsp. chia seed gel (combine a tablespoon of chia seeds with a little water and leave for a few minutes to form gel)

1 tbsp. coconut oil

1 cup filtered water or coconut water

Directions

1. Pulse all the ingredients in your blender until you achieve a smooth consistency.
2. Serve in a tall glass.
3. Enjoy!

Green tea Breakfast Smoothie

Ingredients

½ cup unsweetened green tea, cold

1 ripe banana

1 cup almond milk

Stevia, to taste

Crushed ice

Directions

1. Combine all the ingredients in your blender and pulse until smooth. This is the perfect breakfast smoothie for those days you are feeling like crawling back to bed though you need to go work. Enjoy!

Coconut-Almond-Date Smoothie

Ingredients

1 can coconut milk

5 large Medjool dates

½ cup raw almonds

Directions

1. Roughly chop the dates and the almonds.
2. Put the coconut milk in the blender and switch it on.
3. Slowly drop in the dates and almonds, and continue blending until it is very smooth. Serve chilled.

Ginger-Pomegranate Smoothie

Ingredients

1 cup pure, organic pomegranate juice, unsweetened

½ cup non-fat Greek yogurt

1/4" fresh ginger root

1 frozen banana

½ cup crushed ice or 4 ice cubes

Directions

1. Blend all the ingredients in your blender and serve.
2. Enjoy!

Green Fruit Smoothie

Ingredients

1 can coconut milk

1 cup packed spinach

1 cup berries (any kind)

½ banana

1 tbsp ground flax seeds

Directions

1. Put all ingredients in the blender.
2. Blend on high until smooth.
3. Serve chilled.

Fruity Breakfast Shake

Ingredients

1 cup of blueberries (frozen)

1 banana, fresh or frozen

2 Tablespoons of chia seeds

½ f cup of cold water

1 cup of raspberries (frozen)

1 cup of coconut milk

Directions

1. Combine all the ingredients in an electric blender.

2. Run the blender until all the ingredients are thoroughly blended and it becomes a smoothie.

3. Serve and drink immediately!

Chai Breakfast Smoothie

Ingredients

1 ½ cups almond milk or coconut milk

1 chai tea bag

½ cup pumpkin puree

1 tsp vanilla extract

1 scoop chocolate protein powder

Ice cubes

A handful of cacao nibs

Directions

1. Mix all the ingredients in a blender apart from the cacao nibs and pulse until silky smooth.

2. Serve the smoothie in a tall glass, reserve the rest and top with a generous sprinkle of cacao nibs.

3. Enjoy!

Mixed Berry Smoothie

Ingredients

1 cup black berries

1 cup straw berries

1 cup blue berries

1 medium banana

1 tsp. honey

¾ coconut milk

Directions

1. Slice the banana and combine with all the other ingredients in a blender until you achieve the desired consistency.

Creamy Chia Blueberry Smoothie

Ingredients

½ avocado

½ cup frozen blueberries

½ frozen banana

¼ tsp cinnamon

1 tbsp. chia seed gel (combine a tablespoon of chia seeds with a little water and leave for a few minutes to form gel)

1 tbsp. coconut oil

1 cup filtered water or coconut water

Directions

1. Pulse all the ingredients in your blender until you achieve a smooth consistency.

2. Serve in a tall glass.

3. Enjoy!

Creamy Green Smoothie

Ingredients

1 cup canned coconut milk

½ banana, frozen

1 cup of fresh spinach

½ avocado, pitted

4 pitted medjool dates

1/2 tsp. cinnamon

Directions

1. Place all ingredients into a high speed blender, and blend until smooth.

2. Serve right away. You can enjoy this as a smoothie through a straw, or even as a smoothie bowl.

Delicious Protein Breakfast Smoothie

Ingredients:

3 Tbsp. hemp seeds

1 cup frozen pineapple

2 cups spinach

1 Tbsp. chia seeds

2 cups Almond milk

Directions

1. Add all the ingredients to a high speed blender and mix until done.

2. Pour into a glass and enjoy.

Breakfast Recipes

Berry breakfast bowl

Ingredients

½ cup strawberries

½ cup blackberries

½ cup raspberries

½ cup blueberries

1/8 -1/4 cup cooked quinoa

10 whole toasted almonds, roughly chopped

1 ½ tbsp. hemp hearts

Directions

1. Combine all the ingredients in a large bowl and toss well until evenly combined.
2. Divide the mixture into two bowls and top with a dollop of non-fat Greek yogurt for a protein punch.
3. Yum!

Blueberry quinoa power breakfast muffins

Ingredients

1 cup oatmeal

1 cup cooked quinoa, cooled

1/4 cup raw brown sugar

¼ cup natural honey

1/3 cup flaxseed

1 tsp baking soda

1 tsp baking powder

2 tsp cinnamon

1 cup fresh/ frozen blueberries

1 tsp pure vanilla extract

½ cup organic applesauce

¾ cup non-fat plain Greek yogurt

Directions

1. Start by setting your oven to 350F and prepare a baking tin by lightly greasing it using non-stick cooking spray.
2. In a large bowl, combine all the dry ingredients until evenly combined then set aside. In a separate bowl, whisk together all the wet ingredients until

you get an even consistency. Make a well in the dry ingredients and pour in the wet ingredients.

3. Mix the two until well combined but don't overwork the batter, else you will get the toughest muffins. Gently fold in the berries then scoop the batter into the muffin tin, filling each cup about ¾ way full.
4. Bake for about 20 minutes or until an inserted toothpick emerges clean.
5. Remove from oven and cool on a wire rack. Serve warm.
6. Enjoy!

Energizing Acai Bowl

Ingredients

2 organic acai smoothie pack, frozen

2/3 cup coconut milk, reduced fat

1 ripe frozen banana

¼ cup frozen blueberries

Toppings:

Chopped walnuts/ almonds

Fresh blue berries

1 tsp shredded coconut, unsweetened

1 tsp cacao nibs

1 tsp goji berries

Directions

1. Combine the smoothie packs, frozen fruit and coconut milk in a blender and pulse until smooth and creamy.
2. Pour the smoothie in a bowl and top with all the toppings. Yum!

Smoked salmon-egg white sandwich

Ingredients

30g smoked salmon

2 large egg whites, lightly beaten

1 tbsp. finely chopped Vidalia onion

1 tomato, sliced

½ tsp extra virgin olive oil

½ tsp capers, rinsed and finely chopped

1 whole wheat English muffin, halved and toasted

Salt to taste

Directions

1. Add the olive oil to a small pan over medium heat and sauté the onion until soft for a minute or so. Add the egg whites, capers and salt and cook for about 30 seconds until the whites set.
2. To assemble the sandwich, layer the eggs, salmon and tomato slices on the toasted English muffin.
3. Serve with freshly squeezed orange juice.
4. Enjoy!

Cherry-nut oatmeal

Ingredients

½ cup old-fashioned rolled oats

2 tbsp. dried tart cherries, chopped

1 cup water

1 ½ tbsp. toasted walnuts, chopped

1 tbsp. low fat cream cheese

½ tsp fresh lemon zest

1 tsp natural honey, or to taste

A pinch of salt

Directions

1. Bring the water to a boil over medium heat and add a pinch of salt. Add in the oats and cook for 5 minutes over medium-low heat. Remove from heat and let stand, covered, for 3 minutes.
2. Serve on a bowl and top with the cherries, nuts, lemon zest, cheese and honey.
3. Yum!

Healthy herbed frittata

Ingredients

3 free range eggs, beaten

1 tsp extra virgin olive oil

¼ cup water

1 cup finely diced onion

2 tsp. freshly chopped mixed fresh herbs (dill, parsley, chervil and marjoram)

2 tbsp. low fat farmer's cheese

Salt to taste

Freshly ground black pepper to taste

Directions

1. Add the water to a small nonstick pan over medium-high heat and add in the diced onion. Bring to a boil and cook, covered for 2 minutes. Uncover and continue cooking for about 2 minutes until all the water evaporates.
2. Pour in the olive oil and cook the onions until they start browning for another 2 minutes or so.
3. Pour in the eggs and cook while stirring constantly using a rubber spatula. Lift the edges so the uncooked egg flows underneath.
4. When the egg is almost set, lower the heat and sprinkle the pepper, herbs and salt. Top with the cheese and gently lift the eggs and add a tablespoon of water beneath it.
5. Cover and cook for 2 minutes and serve hot.
6. Enjoy!

Breakfast Fruit Salad

This salad provides a mix of everything you need to give you a balanced start for the day. You can make this the night before to have it ready for breakfast the next morning.

Ingredients

1 banana

1 mango

1 cup berries (any kind)

½ cup cashews

squeeze of lemon

Directions

1. Peel the banana and cut into ½-inch coins.

2. Peel the mango and chop into small cubes.

3. Combine with the berries and cashews, and squeeze a bit of lemon over the salad.

Apple & Sweet Potato Pancakes

Ingredients

1 Tablespoon of agave nectar

3 medium sized sweet potatoes

1 granny smith apple

1 teaspoon of sea salt

8 Tablespoons of coconut flour

1 teaspoon of vanilla essence

2 teaspoons of ground cinnamon, divided

6 pastured eggs

1 teaspoon of baking powder

Coconut oil, as required to fry the pancakes

2 Tablespoons of ghee

Directions

1. Peel the sweet potato and cut into one inch cubes

2. Peel the apple and chop it finely.

3. Take a skillet and put the ghee in it along with a teaspoon of ground cinnamon.

4. Set the flame to medium heat.

5. Cook till ghee is completely melted and hot, then put the chopped apples in it.

6. Cook and stir until the apples are tender. When the apples are soft, take out and set aside.

7. Now take a large saucepan and fill it with water.

8. Put about half teaspoon salt in the water.

9. Bring the water to a boil.

10. When the water is boiling, put the sweet potatoes in it.

11. Boil for 10 - 15 minutes, until the sweet potatoes are tender.

12. Drain the sweet potatoes and set them aside.

13. Now take a mixing bowl and place the coconut flour in it along with the sea salt, baking powder and the remaining one teaspoon of ground cinnamon. Mix well and set aside.

14. Take a food processor and place the sweet potatoes in it.

15. Run the processor till the potatoes take the form of a puree.

16. Put the vanilla extract, pastured eggs and agave nectar in the processor.

17. Run the processor again until all the ingredients are well combined.

18. Now put the coconut flour mixture in the processor.

19. Run the processor till the flour is thoroughly combined with all the other ingredients.

20. Take a griddle or frying pan and put about a teaspoon of oil in it.

21. When the oil is hot, put about a cup of pancake batter in it.

22. Fry the pancake over medium low flame. When one side is brown, flip and brown the other side.

23. Likewise, fry all the other pancakes.

24. Serve the pancakes with apple-cinnamon mixture.

Sweet Potato & Bacon Stir Fry

Ingredients

3 sweet potatoes

5 seitan bacon strips, cubed

1 small red onion, finely chopped

1 clove garlic, minced

¼ tsp. salt

½ tsp. all-spice

1 tbsp. olive oil

Directions

1. Boil the sweet potatoes, aldente

2. Peel the potatoes and cut them into cubes

3. In a wok, pour the oil and place over medium heat. Add the sietan and fry until crispy. Remove the seitan and put in a plate and crush into even smaller pieces.

4. Add the onion and garlic into the wok until the onions are slightly browned then pour in the crushed bacon. Mix a little and add salt and the all-spice. Stir them together and add the cubed sweet potatoes. Keep on turning for about 10 minutes and you are ready to serve.

5. Enjoy!

Breakfast Sausage and Mushroom Casserole

Ingredients

450g of Italian sausage, cooked and crumbled

Three-fourth cup of coconut milk

8 ounces of white mushrooms, sliced

1 medium onion, finely diced

2 Tablespoons of organic ghee

6 free range eggs

600g of sweet potatoes

1 red bell pepper, roasted

3/4 teaspoon of ground black pepper, divided

1 ½ teaspoon of sea salt, divided

Directions

1. Peel and shred the sweet potatoes.

2. Take a bowl, fill it with ice cold water and soak the sweet potatoes in it. Set aside.

3. Peel the roasted bell pepper, remove its seeds and finely dice it.

4. Set the oven to preheat to 375 degrees Fahrenheit.

5. Take a casserole baking dish and grease it with the organic ghee.

6. Put a skillet over medium flame and cook the mushrooms in it. Cook until the mushrooms are crispy and brown.

7. Take the mushrooms out and mix them with the crumbled sausage.

8. Now sauté the onions in the same skillet. Cook till the onions are soft and golden. This should take about 4 – 5 minutes.

9. Take the onions out and mix them in the sausage-mushroom mixture.

10. Add the diced bell pepper to the same mixture. Mix well and set aside for a while.

11. Now drain the soaked shredded potatoes, put them on a paper towel and pat dry.

12. Put the sweet potatoes in a bowl and add about a teaspoon of salt and half a teaspoon of ground black pepper to it. Mix well and set aside.

13. Now take a large bowl and crack the eggs in it.

14. Whisk the eggs and then blend in the coconut milk.

15. Stir in the remaining black pepper and salt.

16. Take the greased casserole dish and spread evenly the seasoned sweet potatoes in the base of the dish.

17. Next, spread evenly the sausage mixture in the dish.

18. Finally, spread the egg mixture.

19. Now cover the casserole dish using a piece of aluminium foil.

20. Bake for 20 - 30 minutes. To check if the casserole is baked properly, insert a tester in the middle of the casserole and it should come out clean.

21. Uncover the casserole dish and bake it again, uncovered for 5 - 10 minutes, until the casserole is a little golden on the top.

22. Allow it to cool for 10 minutes.

23. Enjoy!

Yummy Steak Muffins

Ingredients

1 cup of finely diced red bell pepper

2 Tablespoons of water

8 ounce thin steak, cooked and finely chopped

¼ teaspoon of sea salt

Dash of freshly ground black pepper

8 free range eggs

1 cup of finely diced onion

Directions

1. Set the oven to preheat at 350 degrees Fahrenheit.
2. Take 8 muffin tins and line then with parchment paper liners.
3. Take a large bowl and crack all the eggs in it.
4. Beat well the eggs.
5. Blend in all the remaining ingredients.
6. Scoop out the batter into the prepared muffin tins. Fill three-fourth of each tin.
7. Put the muffin tins in the preheated oven for about 20 minutes, until the muffins are baked and set in the middle.
8. Enjoy!

Coconut Muffins

Ingredients

½ cup of coconut flour

1 teaspoon of baking soda

½ cup of cacao chips

1 teaspoon of sea salt

Stevia to taste

1 cup of almond milk

1 cup of almond flour

6 large free range eggs

½ cup of melted coconut oil

½ cup of chopped mixed nuts

Directions

1. Set the oven to preheat to 350 degrees Fahrenheit.

2. Take 12 muffin tins and line then with parchment paper liners.

3. Take a large bowl and combine coconut flour, baking soda, sea salt, almond flour and mixed nuts in it. Mix well.

4. Stir in the eggs.

5. Blend in the stevia, coconut milk and almond milk and cacao chips. Blend well.

6. Scoop out the batter into the prepared muffin tins. Fill three-fourth of each tin.

7. Put the muffin tins in the preheated oven for about 20 minutes. To check if the muffins are baked properly, insert a tester in the middle of a muffin and it should come out clean.

8. Enjoy!

White and Green Quiche

Ingredients

3 cups of fresh spinach, chopped

15 large free range eggs

3 cloves of garlic, minced

5 white mushrooms, sliced

1 small sized onion, finely chopped

1 ½ teaspoons of baking powder

Ground black pepper to taste

1 ½ cups of coconut milk

Ghee, as required to grease the dish

Sea salt to taste

Directions

1. Set the oven to preheat to 350 degrees Fahrenheit.

2. Take a baking dish and grease it with the organic ghee.

3. Crack all the eggs in a large bowl and whisk well.

4. Stir in coconut milk. Beat well

5. While you are whisking the eggs, start adding the remaining ingredients in it.

6. When all the ingredients are thoroughly blended, pour all of it into the prepared baking dish.

7. Bake for 40 minutes, or until the quiche is set in the middle.Enjoy!

Deviled Eggs

Ingredients

4 hardboiled eggs

1 tsp whole-grain mustard (check ingredients)

2 tbsp Homemade Mayonnaise

pinch salt and black pepper

½ tsp paprika

Directions

1. Peel the hardboiled eggs and cut them carefully in half. Set the whites on a plate and put the yolks into a small bowl.

2. Add the mustard, mayonnaise, salt, and pepper. Mash with a fork until it forms a smooth paste.

3. Using a small spoon, scoop a bit of the yolk mixture into each white. Sprinkle each half with paprika and serve right away or store in the fridge.

Delicious Spicy Pumpkin Patties

Serves: 8

Serving Size: 2 patties

INGREDIENTS

4 cups pumpkin puree

½ cup kale, chopped

½ cup almond meal

1 tablespoon chia seeds

1 tablespoon sesame seeds

2 eggs, lightly beaten

1 teaspoon sea salt

1 teaspoon pepper

1 teaspoon crushed red pepper

½ teaspoon cumin

1 teaspoon turmeric

1 tablespoon coconut oil

Instructions:

1. Preheat oven to 350 degrees Fahrenheit.

2. Heat the coconut oil in a large pan over medium-high heat. Cook the kale until crispy.

3. In a medium bowl, mix the pumpkin puree with the almond meal, chia seed and sesame seeds. Stir in the spices.

4. Fold the eggs and cooked kale into the pumpkin mixture.

5. Drop heaping tablespoons of the pumpkin mixture onto a baking sheet that has been sprayed with non-stick spray.

6. Bake for 30 minutes, or until the patties are firm and golden brown.

7. Serve warm.

The pumpkin in this savory breakfast is high in fiber, while the eggs provide protein, both of which help to keep your appetite at bay.

Apple & Cinnamon Porridge

Serves: 4

Serving Size: 6 ounces

INGREDIENTS

½ cup whole cashews

½ cup whole almonds

¼ cup walnuts

1/3 cup unsweetened coconut flakes

1 large, ripe banana

1 tablespoon coconut oil

1 medium apple, chopped

¼ teaspoon nutmeg

1 teaspoon cinnamon

1 teaspoon vanilla extract

1 (14 ounce can) coconut milk

Instructions:

1. Add the nuts and coconut flakes to a medium bowl. Cover with water and soak 7-8 hours or overnight.

2. Drain the soaked nuts/coconut and rinse well. Add to a food processor along with the banana.

3. Pulse the mixture until a fine meal forms. Scraping down the sides, as needed.

4. Add the coconut oil to a saucepan over medium heat. Add the chopped apple, cinnamon, and nutmeg. Cook until softened.

5. Stir in the coconut milk and vanilla extract. Then add the nut mixture.

6. Bring to a gentle simmer and allow to cook for 5 minutes, or until thick and creamy.

7. Ladle into bowls and top with a splash of almond milk.

Heart healthy nuts take the place of grains in this warming breakfast. Nuts are a good source of unsaturated fats, which have been shown to help lower cholesterol levels.

Baked Eggs

Ingredients

4 eggs

1 tsp extra-virgin olive oil

1 cup cherry tomatoes

2 cups spinach

1 cup mushrooms

2 slices ham (optional)

pinch salt and pepper

Directions

1. Preheat the oven to 450°F and rub a small baking dish with the olive oil.

2. Halve the tomatoes, slice the mushrooms, and roughly chop the ham and spinach. Scatter all of them on the bottom of the baking dish,

3. Crack the eggs carefully on top of the vegetables, then season with salt and pepper. Bake for 8-10 minutes, until the whites are set.

Yummy Zucchini Latkes

Ingredients

2 medium zucchini, shredded(use a clean towel to squeeze out extra moisture from the shredded zucchini)

1 large sweet potato, peeled and shredded

1 tbsp. coconut flour

1 tbsp. coconut oil or ghee

1 tbsp. extra virgin olive oil

1 free range egg, lightly beaten

¼ tsp cumin

2 tsp fresh parsley, minced

½ tsp garlic powder

Kosher salt

Freshly ground pepper

Directions

1. Mix the shredded veggies, minced parsley and the beaten egg in a bowl then set aside. In a separate bowl, combine all the dry ingredients then add this mixture to the veggie bowl and combine well until all the ingredients are well blended.

2. Now, heat the coconut oil and olive oil in a non-stick skillet.

3. Drop about a fifth of the 'batter' into the skillet and press down to form a latke using a fork and cook until crisp and golden, for about 2 minutes per side. Transfer to a plate lined with paper towels and repeat the process for the remaining batter.

4. To serve, sprinkle with a bit of kosher salt. Enjoy!

Turkey Breakfast Scramble

Ingredients

1 pound ground lean turkey

1 cup of mushrooms, sliced

1 onion, chopped

½ teaspoon salt

½ teaspoon Italian seasoning

2 tablespoons French style mustard

1/2 cup of fresh basil to garnish

2 Tbsp. coconut oil for cooking

Directions

1. Heat the coconut oil in a large skillet over medium heat, and cook the mushrooms with the onions for 4 minutes

2. -Once the mushrooms, and onions are cooked, season with the salt, and Italian seasoning.

3. -Set the vegetables aside, and cook the ground lean turkey in the same pan over medium heat with an additional tablespoon of coconut oil, cook until the turkey is cooked all the way through.

4. -Once the turkey is cooked, combine the ground turkey with the mushroom, and onion, and mix in the French mustard.

5. -Spoon the scramble onto 4 serving dishes, and garnish with the fresh basil.

Pork and Egg Breakfast Casserole

Ingredients

1 Tablespoon of olive oil

Pinch of ground black pepper

2 Tablespoons of chopped basil

16 ounces of pork tenderloin, shredded

8 large free range eggs, scrambled

1 medium red onion, diced

1 cup of finely diced zucchini

3 cloves of garlic, chopped

Pinch of sea salt

Organic ghee, as required to grease the baking dish

Directions

1. Set the oven to preheat to 350 degrees Fahrenheit.
2. Take a casserole baking dish and grease it with the organic ghee.
3. Heat oil in a skillet and turn on the flame to medium high.
4. Sauté the onions and garlic in it. Cook till the onions are caramelized.
5. Take the onions and garlic out of the skillet. Set aside.

6. Crack the eggs in a bowl and whisk well.

7. Stir in the zucchini, basil, salt, pork and pepper. Beat well

8. Whisk in the caramelized onion and garlic.

9. Pour the entire mixture evenly into the prepared casserole dish.

10. Bake for 30 minutes, or until the casserole is set in the middle.

11. Relocate the casserole dish and place it directly under the broiler.

12. Bake for about 5 minutes, until the casserole is lightly brown at the top.

13. Enjoy!

Zucchini and Steak Casserole

Ingredients

250g steak, cooked then shredded

3 large sized zucchinis, grated

1 teaspoon of sea salt

5 free range eggs

Ground black pepper, to taste

Half Tablespoon of olive oil

1 small red onion, finely diced

Directions

1. Set the oven to preheat to 375 degrees Fahrenheit.

2. Take an oven-safe skillet and heat it over medium flame.

3. Crack the eggs in a bowl and beat well along with salt and pepper.

4. Take about large bowl and combine all the remaining ingredients in it. Mix well.

5. Stir in the shredded steak.

6. Stir in the eggs.

7. Heat the olive oil in an oven-safe skillet over medium flame.

8. When the oil is hot, add the zucchini mixture to it.

9. Cover the pan and let it cook for five minutes.

10. Turn off the flame and transfer the skillet to the preheated oven.

11. Bake for 10 - 15 minutes, till the eggs are cooked and firm.

12. Take the skillet out of the oven and let sit for 10 minutes.

13. Enjoy!

Beef Breakfast Casserole

Ingredients

1 pound of ground beef, cooked

10 eggs

½ cup Pico de Gallo

1 cup baby spinach

¼ cup sliced black olives

Freshly ground black pepper

Directions

1. Preheat oven to 350 degrees Fahrenheit. Prepare a 9" glass pie plate with non-stick spray.

2. Whisk the eggs until frothy. Season with salt and pepper.

3. Layer the cooked ground beef, Pico de Gallo, and spinach in the pie plate.

4. Slowly pour the eggs over the top.

5. Top with black olives.

6. Bake for 30 minutes, until firm in the middle.

7. Slice into 5 pieces and serve.

"Toast" Negative Calorie Style

Ingredients:

2 large sweet potato cooked with skin on, and sliced into 4 large strips to be used s "toast"

1 avocado

4 fried eggs

Pinch of cayenne pepper

Salt to taste

Directions

1. After the sweet potatoes are cooked, and sliced into large bread like strips, top each sweet potato strip with sliced avocado, and 1 egg each.

2. Season with a small pinch of cayenne pepper to add some heat, and sea salt to taste.

3. 2 slices per serving.

Breakfast Bowl

Ingredients:

1 egg cooked over easy

1 mashed banana

1/2 of an apple, chopped into cubes

1 Tbsp. of almond butter

1/2 Tbsp. of shredded coconut

1 tsp. of cinnamon

Directions

1. Place the cooked egg, and mashed banana at the bottom of a bowl.

2. Top with the apple, almond butter, coconut, and cinnamon.

Chocolate Banana Bowl

Ingredients

1 sliced banana

1/2 cup of fresh berries of choice

1 Tbsp. of dark cocoa nibs (Unsweetened)

1 Tbsp. almond butter

1 Tbsp. sliced almonds

Directions

1. Place the sliced banana at the bottom of a cereal bowl, and top with all of the yummy toppings.

Ham and Veggie Frittata Muffins

Serves: 12

Serving Size: 1 muffin

Ingredients:

5 ounces thinly sliced ham

8 large eggs

4 tablespoons coconut oil

½ yellow onion, finely diced

8 oz. frozen spinach, thawed and drained

8 oz. mushrooms, thinly sliced

1 cup cherry tomatoes, halved

¼ cup coconut milk (canned)

2 tablespoons coconut flour

Sea salt and pepper to taste

Directions

1. Preheat oven to 375 degrees Fahrenheit.

2. In a medium skillet, melt the coconut oil over medium heat. Add the onion and cook until softened.

3. Add the mushrooms, spinach and cherry tomatoes. Season with salt and pepper. Cook until the

mushrooms have softened. About 5 minutes.
Remove from heat and set aside.

4. In a large bowl whisk the eggs together with the
    coconut milk and coconut flour. Stir in the cooled
    the veggie mixture.

5. Line each cavity of a 12 cavity muffin tin with the
    thinly sliced ham. Pour the egg mixture into each
    one and bake for 20 minutes.

6. Remove from oven and allow to cool for about 5
    minutes before transferring to a wire rack.

*To maximize the benefit of a vegetable rich diet, it's
important to eat a variety of colors and these veggie
packed frittata muffins do just that. The onion, spinach,
mushrooms, and cherry tomatoes provide a wide range of
vitamin and nutrients as well as a healthy dose of fiber.*

Tomato and Avocado Omelet

Serves: 1

Serving Size: 1 omelet

Ingredients

2 eggs

¼ avocado, diced

4 cherry tomatoes, halved

1 tablespoon cilantro, chopped

Squeeze of lime juice

Pinch of salt

Directions

1. In a small bowl, combine the avocado, tomatoes, cilantro, lime juice and salt. Mix well and set aside.

2. Heat a medium, nonstick skillet over medium heat. Whisk the eggs until frothy and add to the pan. Move the eggs around gently with a rubber spatula until they begin to set.

3. Scatter the avocado mixture over half of the omelet. Remove from heat, and slide the omelet onto a plate as you fold it in half.

4. Serve immediately.

Egg Stuffed Sweet Potatoes

Serves: 2

Serving Size: 1 sweet potato + 2 eggs

Ingredients

2 medium sweet potatoes

4 eggs

4 slices bacon

1 small yellow onion, diced

4 cloves garlic, minced

Sea salt and pepper

Directions

1. Preheat oven to 400 degrees Fahrenheit. Bake sweet potatoes for about 40-45 minutes, until soft. Remove from oven and allow to cool.

2. In a large skillet, cook the bacon until crisp. Remove from pan and add the onion and garlic. Cook for about 5-7 minutes, until translucent.

3. Cut the sweet potatoes in half lengthwise and scoop out the flesh. Add to the pan with the onion and garlic. Season with salt and pepper. Chop the bacon and add to the sweet potato mixture.

4. Place the sweet potato skins onto a baking sheet and fill each with the mixture.

5. Make a small divot in each and crack an egg into it.

6. Cook for 15 minutes, or until the yolk is set.

7. Enjoy immediately!

Sweet potatoes are surprisingly low on the glycemic index and contain high amounts of fiber, potassium, and several vitamins, especially vitamin A. And while they do contain carbs and natural sugar, they have minimal effects on blood sugar levels because of their high fiber content.

Fiesta Egg Muffins

Serves: 12

Serving Size: 1 muffin

Ingredients

1 tablespoon olive oil

2 bell peppers (any color), diced

1 small red onion, diced

3 green onions, sliced

1 tomato, diced

¼ cup salsa

12 eggs

Sea salt and pepper to taste

Directions

1. Preheat oven to 350 degrees Fahrenheit.

2. Prepare a cupcake or muffin tin by brushing each cavity with olive oil.

3. Heat the olive oil in a skillet over medium-high heat. Sauté the onions and peppers until soft. Add the tomato and green onion and cook for another minute. Divide the vegetable mixture evenly into each cavity of the muffin tin.

4. Whisk the eggs until frothy. Stir in the salsa and season with salt and pepper. Pour the egg mixture into the muffin tin.

5. Bake for 15-20 minutes, or until the eggs are set.

6. Allow to cool slightly before removing from the muffin tin with a spoon or butter knife.

7. Enjoy immediately or wrap in plastic wrap and store in the refrigerator or freezer for an easy breakfast on the go.

These fiesta egg muffins are a great make ahead meal. Make 1 or 2 batches of them at the beginning of the week, wrap tightly in plastic wrap and store in the fridge. When you need a quick breakfast or snack on the go, just pop in the microwave to heat up and breakfast is served!

Spicy Sausage Wrapped Eggs

Serves: 6

Serving Size: 2 eggs

Ingredients

12 ounce packages of chorizo sausage

12-ounce package of ground pork

2 teaspoons chili powder (more or less to taste)

3 cloves garlic, minced

12 hard boiled eggs

Directions

1. Preheat oven to 375 degrees Fahrenheit.

2. Combine all of the ingredients except for the eggs in a large bowl and mix well with your hands. Divide the mixture into 12 equal pieces.

3. To wrap the eggs: Lay a piece of plastic wrap down on your work surface. Take one portion of the pork mixture and flatten it out onto the plastic wrap. Place a hard boiled egg in the middle and lift the plastic wrap, wrapping the egg in the sausage mixture. Repeat for all eggs.

4. Place eggs on a baking sheet and bake for 30 minutes, until sausage is cooked through.

5. Can be served warm of cool.

Eggless Mexican Breakfast Bowl

Serves: 2

Serving Size: 1 bowl

Ingredients

1 teaspoon coconut oil

½ small onion, sliced

1 bell pepper, sliced

½ pound ground pork or chicken

½ teaspoon oregano

¼ teaspoon cumin

Sea salt and pepper

1 avocado, mashed

4 tablespoons salsa

Directions

1. In a large skillet, heat the coconut oil over medium heat. Add the onions and pepper to the pan and cook until softened.

2. Once the vegetables are cooked, move them to the side of the pan and add the ground pork. Season with oregano, cumin, salt and pepper.

3. Break the pork into chunks as it cooks and mix well with the onions and peppers.

4. Split the mixture between two bowls and top each with mashed avocado and salsa.

Avocados are a true super food. With health benefits that include weight management, protection from cardiovascular disease, and enhancing the absorption of nutrients to the body, there's no reason not to include them in your meals! Avocados come in many varieties, but the most common is the creamy Haas variety.

Greek Breakfast Casserole

Serves: 5

Ingredients

1 pound of ground chicken, cooked

10 eggs

1 small red onion, thinly sliced

1 cup baby spinach

¼ cup sliced Kalamata olives

½ teaspoon oregano

Freshly ground black pepper

Directions

1. Preheat oven to 350 degrees Fahrenheit. Prepare a 9" glass pie plate with non-stick spray.

2. Whisk the eggs until frothy. Season with oregano and pepper.

3. Layer the cooked ground chicken, red onion, and spinach in the pie plate.

4. Slowly pour the eggs over the top.

5. Top with Kalamata olives.

6. Bake for 30 minutes, until firm in the middle.

7. Slice into 5 pieces and serve.

Breakfast Skillet

Serves: 6

Serving Size: 1 cup + 1 egg

Ingredients

1-pound grass-fed steak, cut into ½" pieces (sirloin works well)

2 medium sweet potatoes, peeled and diced

1 green pepper, diced

1 red bell pepper, diced

1 small yellow onion, diced

2 tablespoons coconut oil

Sea salt and pepper to taste

6 large eggs

1 small tomato, sliced

Directions

1. Preheat oven to 350 degrees Fahrenheit. Melt 1 tablespoon of the coconut oil in a medium skillet over medium heat. Cook the steak until just browned. Set aside.

2. Add the remaining coconut oil to the pan and cook the onion and peppers until softened. Add the sweet potatoes and sauté for about 10 minutes, or until tender.

3. Add the steak back to the pan and stir to combine. Remove from heat and make 6 divots in the mixture.

4. Crack an egg into each divot, place the sliced tomato on top, and season everything with salt and pepper.

5. Bake for 10-12 minutes, or until the eggs are cooked to your liking.

6. Remove from oven and serve immediately.

Grass-fed beef contains two to six times the amount of omega-3 fatty acids than traditional grain fed beef. These omega-3s play a vital role in heart and brain health. Research has also shown that grass-fed beef is four times higher in vitamin E, which has been linked to a lower risk of cancer and heart disease.

Creamy Spinach & Poached Eggs

Serves: 4

Serving Size: 2 eggs + spinach

Ingerdients

4 large eggs

4 cups baby spinach

2 teaspoons coconut oil

2 cloves garlic, minced

2 tablespoons coconut cream

Sea salt and pepper to taste

Directions

1. In a large skillet, heat the coconut oil over medium heat. Add the garlic and sauté until it starts to brown. Increase heat to medium high and add the baby spinach. Season with salt and pepper and cook until wilted.

2. Remove from heat and stir in the coconut cream.

3. Meanwhile, heat a saucepan of water to simmering and poach your eggs.

4. When the eggs are cooked, divide the spinach onto 2 plates and use the back of a spoon to make a well in the spinach.

5. Slide the eggs onto the spinach and serve!

Egg poaching tip: Add a few tablespoons of vinegar to gently simmering water – it will help to hold the egg whites together. 4 minutes will give you firm egg whites with a soft yolk. Leave it in a minute longer and you'll have a yolk that's custardy and soft.

Ham & Broccoli Frittata

Serves: 6

Serving Size: 1 slice

Ingredients

2 tablespoons coconut oil

½ yellow onion, diced

10 oz. ham, cubed

1 ½ cups broccoli, chopped into small pieces

10 eggs

½ cup coconut milk

½ teaspoon salt

¼ teaspoon pepper

¼ teaspoon garlic powder

¼ teaspoon crushed red pepper

Directions

1. Preheat oven to 400 degrees Fahrenheit.

2. Heat the coconut oil in a large skillet over medium-high heat. Sauté the ham and onion until golden, about 7-8 minutes. Add the broccoli and continue cooking for 2-3 minutes.

3. In a large bowl, whisk together the eggs, coconut milk, and spices. Pour into the skillet and transfer to oven.

4. Bake for 20 minutes, or until the eggs are puffy and golden brown.

5. Let rest for 5-10 minutes before slicing and serving.

Broccoli has a strong, positive impact on our body's detoxification system, ridding the body of unwanted contaminates while helping to neutralize PH levels.

Lunch Recipes

Zesty Chicken Bites

Serves: 3-4

Serving Size: 6-7 chicken bites

Ingredients

1 pound skinless, boneless chicken breasts

1 egg

¼ cup water

¾ cup almond meal

2 teaspoons Italian seasoning

½ teaspoon cayenne pepper

½ teaspoon paprika

1 teaspoon garlic powder

½ teaspoon crushed red pepper

½ teaspoon chili powder (can be adjusted to desired level of spiciness)

½ teaspoon sea salt

Directions

1. Preheat oven to 400 degrees. Prepare a metal baking sheet with non-stick spray.

2. In a medium bowl combine the almond meal and spices. Mix well.

3. In a separate bowl, whisk the egg and water together.

4. Cut the chicken into bite sized pieces.

5. Drop the chicken into the egg mixture, then transfer to the spice mixture.

6. Place the chicken pieces on the prepared baking sheet. Bake for 25-30 minutes, flipping halfway through, until the chicken is crispy and golden brown.

7. Serve immediately and store any leftovers in an airtight container in the refrigerator.

Chicken is an important staple in any whole food diet. It's a low-fat form of protein and its versatility cannot be matched. Chicken's high vitamin B6 content has been shown to boost metabolism and keep energy levels high.

A veggie extravaganza!

Ingredients

1 cup celery, diced

2 cups baby spinach

1 cup cauliflower florets

2 cups shredded cabbage

1 cup green beans, cut into 1 inch pieces

2 cups diced zucchini

1 onion, diced

1 cup diced turnip

1 jalapeno, seeded and finely chopped

3 cloves garlic, finely grated

Salt to taste

Freshly ground pepper to taste

6 cups low sodium vegetable stock – preferably home-made

Directions

1. Combine all the ingredients in a large sauce pan or soup pot except for the baby spinach and place over medium to high heat.

2. Once it comes to a boil, reduce the heat to low and simmer for about 20 minutes, covered.

3. Adjust the seasonings if desired then stir in the baby spinach and cook or 30 seconds to one minute.

4. Serve into soup bowls.

5. Enjoy!

Green Bean Salad with Walnuts

Serves: 3-4

Serving Size: About 1 cup

INGREDIENTS

1 pound fresh green beans, washed, ends snipped, and cut in half

1 red onion, chopped

1 cup walnuts, toasted and chopped

Dressing:

2 tablespoons macadamia nut oil

2 tablespoons olive oil

4 tablespoons Dijon mustard (non-alcoholic option)

4 tablespoons balsamic vinegar

¼ teaspoon garlic powder

¼ teaspoon onion powder

¼ teaspoon sea salt

¼ teaspoon black pepper

Directions

1. Steam green beans until tender. About 5-10 minutes should get them tender, but not mushy.

2. When done steaming, submerge in an ice bath to stop the cooking process and retain their color.

3. In a large bowl, whisk together the dressing ingredients. Add the chopped red onion and stir.

4. Remove the green beans from the water bath and drain.

5. Add the beans to the dressing and toss until they are fully coated. This can be made ahead of time and refrigerated for 2-3 days.

6. Just before serving, top with the toasted walnuts.

Research shows that walnut consumption may support brain health and improve cell function. The crunchy, earthy flavored nut contains a good amount of heart healthy omega-3 fats and fiber to keep you satiated.

Avocado Egg Salad

Serves: 2

INGREDIENTS

1 ripe avocado

2 hardboiled eggs

1 small tomato

Small bunch of cilantro (optional)

Juice from one lemon

Sea salt and pepper to taste

Directions

1. Chop the first four ingredients into small pieces.

2. Mix together in a bowl and combine with lemon juice and salt and pepper.

3. Toss until well combined. Serve atop salad greens, baby spinach, or even inside of a hollowed out tomato for a fancy presentation.

Eggs are a very good source of inexpensive, high quality protein. They also have impressive health credentials. The whites are rich sources of selenium, vitamin D while the yoke contain fat soluble vitamins such as A, D, E and K.

Chipotle Chicken Stuffed Sweet Potatoes

Serves: 2

Serving Size: 1 stuffed potato

INGREDIENTS

2 boneless chicken thighs

2 tablespoons olive oil

1 tablespoon smoked paprika

1-2 teaspoons ground chipotle pepper (depending on desired spiciness)

2 teaspoons garlic salt

1 teaspoon black pepper

2 sweet potatoes

1 cup kale, chopped

½ a red bell pepper, chopped

1 tablespoon olive oil

1 tablespoon lemon juice

Sea salt and pepper to taste

Directions

1. Bake sweet potatoes at 350 degrees Fahrenheit for about 45 minutes to an hour. Until tender. Set aside. (This can be done well in advance. Just reheat when ready to serve.)

2. Heat a large skillet to medium-high. Coat the boneless chicken thighs in the 2 tablespoons olive oil and sprinkle with smoked paprika, chipotle, garlic salt, and pepper.

3. Grill for 5-10 minutes per side (depending on the size). Set aside to rest.

4. Chop the kale and red pepper and add to a bowl. Whisk the olive oil, lemon juice, and salt and pepper together in a small bowl. Add to the kale and massage in, to soften the kale.

5. Finely chop the cooked chicken and add to the kale mixture.

6. To assemble, slice the sweet potato lengthwise and mash the insides slightly. Scoop the chicken/kale mixture into the middle of each sweet potato.

7. Serve immediately or store in an airtight container in the refrigerator.

The kale and chicken stuffing for the sweet potatoes is a great item to make ahead and have on hand for easy lunches. Bake off a tray of sweet potatoes while you've got that going, and your set for the week!

Squash Salad

Ingredients

4 Tablespoons of finely diced red onion

1 cup of finely diced red pepper

Half cup of whole 30 friendly Dijon mustard

1 cup of chopped tomatoes

12 ounces smoked sausage, chopped

1 spaghetti squash, cooked

Directions

1. Take a large serving bowl and place all the ingredients in it.
2. Mix well.
3. Serve!

Mexican Romaine Salad

Ingredients

4 boneless and skinless chicken breasts (8 oz. each)

2 medium onions, sliced

8 Tablespoons of fresh cilantro

1 cup of salad greens

2 cups of homemade guacamole

4 red bell peppers, sliced

1 cups of shredded Romaine

4 Tablespoons of Extra virgin olive oil

Sea salt to taste

Ground black pepper to taste

Directions

1. Season the chicken breasts liberally with salt and pepper. Set aside for a while.

2. Taka a cast iron skillet and heat olive oil in it.

3. When the oil is hot, cook the chicken in it, until it is well done.

4. Take the chicken out of the skillet and set aside.

5. Put the diced onions and bell peppers in the same skillet.

6. Sauté the vegetables over medium high flame.

7. When the onions are soft yet crispy and the pepper is slightly charred, turn off the flame.

8. Cut the cooked chicken breasts into small strips and add them to the vegetables. Mix well.

9. Just before serving, divide the chicken mixture equally on to the serving plates.

10. Garnish each serving of salad with one cup of shredded romaine, and servings of guacamole and salad greens.

11. Finally, top up each serving with about two Tablespoons of chopped cilantro.

12. Enjoy!

Mediterranean Grilled Vegetables

Ingredients

2 eggplants

2 zucchini

2 red bell peppers

2 large portabella mushroom caps

4 leaves fresh basil

½ tsp dried thyme

½ tsp dried oregano

2 tbsp extra-virgin olive oil

2 tbsp balsamic vinegar

Directions

1. Slice the eggplants and zucchini into ½-inch slices. Cut the tops off of the bell peppers, knock out any remaining seeds, and cut them into quarters. Leave the mushrooms whole. Place in a large bowl.

2. Mix the oil, vinegar, and spices together in a small bowl and pour it over the vegetables. Toss to coat, and allow to marinate for 1-2 hours.

3. Preheat the grill to medium-high. Arrange the vegetables on it, with the peppers and eggplants in the hottest parts. Grill until the vegetables are softened and show dark brown grill marks, 10-20 minutes.

Turkish Salad with Pomegranate Molasses

This tangy, fresh salad is a great accompaniment to rich main dishes like lamb or beef.

Ingredients

1 tomato

½ mild white onion

1 bag arugula

1 tbsp olive oil

1 tbsp pomegranate molasses

salt and pepper

Directions

1. Finely dice the tomato and onion. Divide the arugula between two plates and put the vegetables on top. Drizzle with the oil and molasses and sprinkle with salt and pepper.

2. Note: Pomegranate molasses is just pomegranate juice boiled down into a thick syrup. You can make it yourself or find it online or in Middle Easter grocery stores. Make sure you find a brand without added sugar.

Green Mango Salad

Ingredients

2 firm green (unripe) mangos

½ lime

pinch cayenne pepper

a few spring cilantro

Directions

1. Peel and grate the green mangos. Chop the cilantro.

2. Place the grated mango in a medium bowl and squeeze the lime over it. Add the cilantro and cayenne pepper and stir. Serve right away or chilled.

Apple Spinach Salad

Ingredients

1 bunch or bag spinach

½ tart apple

½ cup toasted almonds or walnuts

1 cup strawberries or pomegranate seeds (based on the season)

Homemade Apple Cider Vinaigrette

Directions

1. Chop the apple and slice the strawberries, if using.

2. Put the spinach in a large bowl and toss with Apple Cider Vinaigrette, to taste. Add half the fruit and nuts and toss again.

3. Put it on plates or a serving bowl, and top with the remaining fruit and nuts. Serve right away.

4. Note: To make this into a full meal, add a ½ or whole chicken breast, grilled and chopped.

Roasted Carrots with Curried Cashew Sauce

Ingredients

5 large carrots

1 + ½ tsp curry powder

1 tsp extra-virgin olive oil

¼ cup cashew butter

3-4 tbsp water

pinch salt

2 tsp lime juice

Directions

1. Chop the carrots into ½-inch chunks. Toss with just enough olive oil to coat and 1 tsp curry powder.

2. Spread in a single layer in a baking pan and roast until they are starting to get tender and turning brown on the edges.

3. Meanwhile, whisk the cashew butter with ½ tsp curry powder, the lime juice, and salt. Add 2 tbsp water and keep stirring, keep adding water until it reaches a smooth consistency.

4. Divide the cashew sauce on two small plates, and distribute the carrots evenly between them.

Spicy Italian Salad

Ingredients

1 Jalapeno pepper, chopped

1 Italian plum tomato, chopped

1 clove of garlic, minced

2 ripe avocados

Half cup of minced onion

1 Tablespoon of fresh lime juice

1 Tablespoon of chopped fresh cilantro

Kosher salt to taste

Ground black pepper to taste

Directions

1. Peel and avocadoes and remove the pits.
2. Combine the avocados and lime juice in a juice.
3. Using a fork, mash the avocados coarsely.
4. Add all the remaining veggies and ingredients to the mashed avocadoes.
5. Mix well.
6. Enjoy!

Tuna - Watercress Salad

Ingredients

1 Tablespoon of rice vinegar

1 cup of small watercress sprigs

Half teaspoon of ground coriander

1 Tablespoon of olive oil

3 medium sized oranges

Pinch of cayenne pepper

1 lb of tuna steaks (about 1 inch thick)

1 teaspoon of finely minced ginger

Half teaspoon of ground aniseed, divided

Pinch of pepper

Half teaspoon of sea salt, divided

Directions

1. Cut the steak into bite sized chunks.

2. Peel the oranges and remove the white piths.

3. Relocate the rack of the oven fine inches above the broiler, then preheat it to high temperate.

4. Line a broiler pan with a piece of aluminium foil.

5. Now take a large bowl and place the oranges, rice vinegar, olive oil, half of the salt, cayenne pepper,

half of the ground aniseed, ground coriander and ginger in it. Mix well.

6. Add watercress sprigs. Mix well and set aside.

7. Season the steak with remaining salt, pepper and the remaining ground aniseed.

8. Take the aluminium lined broiler and put the seasoned steaks in it.

9. Reduce the broiler's temperature to medium and broil the steak in it.

10. Broil for four minutes per side.

11. Take the steak out in the serving plate.

12. Serve it with the watercress-orange mixture.

13. Enjoy!

Baked Sweet Potato Fries

Ingredients

2 medium sweet potatoes

1 tbsp extra-virgin olive oil

pinch sea salt and black pepper

Directions

1. Preheat the oven to 450°F and position an oven rack in the middle of the oven. Scrub the sweet potatoes and cut them into long narrow pieces. You can do this by cutting them into 12 wedges, or by cutting ½-inch thick slices and then cutting those into ¼-inch wide matchsticks. Either way, aim for evenly cut pieces about ½-inch wide.

2. Put the sweet potatoes into a large baking pan and drizzle the olive oil over them. Sprinkle with salt and pepper, then use your hands to stir them and ensure they are evenly coated with oil.

3. Bake for 20 minutes, then remove from the oven and flip the fries. Return to the oven for another 20 minutes. If they are still too firm in the middle and not nicely brown, flip and return for another 10-20 minutes. When they are done to your liking, remove from the oven and serve hot.

Note: The type of baking pan, as well as oven position, will really affect the cooking rate. Metal and dark pans go faster, glass and insulated pans go slower. Keep an eye on the fries to prevent burning.

Crunchy Kale Salad with Avocado Dressing

Ingredients

1 bunch kale

1 avocado

juice of ½ lemon

1 tbsp extra-virgin olive oil

1 tsp whole-grain mustard

½ apple

½ cup toasted almonds

salt and pepper

Directions

1. Rinse the kale and chop into 1-inch pieces. Place in a large bowl. Chop the apple and the toasted almonds.

2. Mash the avocado with a fork, then combine the avocado, lemon juice, olive oil, mustard, and salt and pepper in a small bowl. Stir until smooth. Add more lemon juice or water as needed to achieve desired consistency.

3. Drizzle the dressing over the kale and top with the apples and almonds.

Roasted Artichoke Hearts with Lemon and Olives

Ingredients

1 jar artichoke hearts

1 tbsp extra-virgin olive oil

2 cloves garlic

1 lemon

1 cup green olives

1 tsp dried oregano

Directions

1. Preheat the oven to 400°F. Mince the garlic and chop the lemon into small pieces. Drain the artichokes.

2. Toss the artichokes, olives, and lemon with the oil, garlic, salt, and oregano. Spread the mixture on a baking sheet and roast for 15-20 minutes, until the artichokes start to turn golden brown on the edges.

Chard Skillet with Eggs

Ingredients

1 large bunch chard

1 tbsp extra-virgin olive oil

2 cloves garlic, minced

chili flakes to taste

2-3 eggs

Directions

1. Wash the chard and trim the bottoms of the stems. Chop it into 1-2 inch pieces. Meanwhile, heat a large skillet over medium-high. You'll need a cover that fits.

2. Add the olive oil to the skillet, then add the garlic and stir for about 30 seconds, until it is fragrant and starts to turn golden brown. Add chili flakes to taste.

3. Add all the chard and stir well. Cook, stirring occasionally, until it has wilted and starts to turn a darker green, 4-5 minutes.

4. With a spoon, make 2 or 3 (however many eggs you are using) wells in the chard. Carefully crack one egg into each.

5. Sprinkle 2 tbsp of water into the skillet to prevent it from burning and to create steam. Cover the skillet.

6. Check the eggs after two minutes, adding more water if necessary. You can gently stir the chard around the eggs if needed. Recover the skillet.

7. The eggs will take from 5-10 minutes to cook, depending on how hot your pan gets and how firm you like your eggs. You can check them by gently pressing the yolks with the back of a spoon to see if they are firm or still runny. Serve right away.

Moroccan-Style Grilled Ground Beef

Ingredients

¾ pound organic 100% grass-fed ground beef

½ onion, finely grated

½ of a small, medium-spicy green pepper, grated

¼ loosely packed cilantro, finely chopped

¼ salt

1 clove garlic, minced

½ cumin

Directions

1. Preheat your grill to high. Mix all ingredients together in a large bowl. Stir with your hands or a spoon until completely combined.

2. Form the mixture into small patties and place on the grill. Cook for about 4 minutes per side, until the meat is fully cooked.

Apple-Walnut Chicken Salad

Ingredients

2 organic pastured chicken breasts

1 clove garlic

1 bay leaf

1 spring thyme

1 apple

¼ cup toasted walnuts

1 stalk celery

2 tsp mustard

2 tbsp Homemade Mayonnaise

Directions

1. Place the chicken in a medium sauce pan and cover with 2 inches of water. Add the garlic, bay leaf, and thyme, and bring the mixture to a boil. Reduce to a very low simmer and cook until the middle of the breast has reached 165°F or until there is no pink meat.
2. Remove from the poaching water and dry with a paper towel. Cut the chicken into ½-inch cubes and set it aside.
3. Core the apple and chop it into ½-inch cubes. Chop the celery into ¼-inch slices. Mix the mustard with the mayonnaise, then combine it with the apple, celery, and chicken. Stir well. Sprinkle with toasted walnuts and serve immediately or store in the fridge.

Charmila (North African–Style Tomato Poached Eggs)

Ingredients

3 tomatoes

½ large onion

1 clove garlic

a few springs cilantro

a few sprigs parsley

¼ tsp salt

4 eggs

Directions

1. Grate the tomatoes and onion. You can also pulse them in a food processor. Roughly chop the herbs and mince the garlic.

2. Heat a skillet over medium-high and add the tomato mixture and garlic. Bring to a boil, then reduce heat and simmer until the it turns a darker red and becomes thicker. Add the herbs and salt and check that the heat is low.

3. Gently crack the eggs into the pan, evenly spaced. Cover the pan and allow the eggs to poach in the tomato mixture. Check it after 2-3 minutes and add water if it gets too dry.

4. The eggs will take 5-7 minutes to cook, depending on how well you like them done. Press the yolks gently with the back of a spoon to see how firm they are. Once the eggs are cooked, serve it right away.

Moroccan Fish Tagine

Ingredients

1 potato

1 red pepper

1 small spicy green pepper

1 large carrot

½ onion

½ cup green olives

1 clove garlic

½ cumin

2 tbsp extra-virgin olive oil

½ pound fresh sardines

¼ tsp salt

Directions

1. Preheat the oven to 425°F. Pour half the olive oil in the bottom of a round baking dish, such as a 9-inch pie pan. Find something that will work as a lid, such as a pie pan.

2. Peel the potato and chop into ½-inch cubes. Dice the peppers and onion into small squares. Peel and chop the carrot. Mince the garlic.

3. Arrange the carrot around the outside edge of the pan. Put the potatoes on the bottom in the middle.

Scatter the onions, peppers, garlic, cumin, and olives evenly on top of the carrots and potatoes.

4. Arrange the sardines in a single layer over the vegetables. Pour in 3 tbsp of water around the edges and sprinkle the salt over the top.

5. Bake for 20-25 minutes, until the potatoes are tender and the fish flakes easily with a fork. Serve piping hot.

Stuffed Acorn Squash with Sage and Thyme

Ingredients

2 acorn squash

½ pound ground organic turkey

1 tbsp ghee or clarified butter

½ onion

1 stalk celery

1 medium carrot

½ tsp dried sage

½ tsp dried thyme

Directions

1. Preheat the oven to 375°F. cut the acorn squash in half and scrape out all the seeds. Coat the cut side lightly with olive oil and place cut side down in a roasting pan. Place in oven. This will speed up the baking process.

2. Finely dice the onion and celery. Peel the carrot and dice finely as well.

3. In a large pan, heat the ghee over medium. Add the onion, carrot, and celery and cook until the vegetables are softened, about 7 minutes.

4. Add the ground turkey and herbs and continue cooking until browned.

5. Take the squash out of the oven and flip them over. Fill each cavity with some of the turkey mixture and return to the oven. Bake until the squash is tender, 30-40 minutes in total.

Grilled Salmon with Citrus Marinade

Ingredients

1 salmon fillet, ¾ to 1 pound

juice and zest of ½ lemon

juice of 1 orange

2 tbsp orange juice concentrate

1 clove garlic, minced

2 tbsp extra-virgin olive oil

¼ tsp black pepper

pinch salt

Directions

1. Place the salmon in a flat pan. Mix all other ingredients together and pour over the salmon, rubbing it into the fish with the back of a spoon. Put the salmon in the fridge and allow to marinate for 1-2 hours.

2. Preheat the grill to high. Take the fish out of the fridge and carefully pour the marinade into a small saucepan. Bring the mixture to a boil and simmer over low while you grill the fish.

3. Place the salmon flesh-side down on the grill. Grill for 5-7 minutes, until grill marks form and the fish releases easily from the grates. Flip and grill for 5-7 more minutes, or until the flesh flakes easily when pressed with a fork.

4. Allow to rest for 10 minutes, then serve warm with the reduced marinade sauce on the side.

Bacon and Vegetable Frittata

Ingredients

4 pieces uncured organic bacon

6 eggs

1 clove garlic, minced

2 cups spinach

1 cup white mushrooms

1 tbsp extra-virgin olive oil

Directions

1. Cook the bacon in the oven or the microwave (these methods greatly reduce the formation of cancer-causing nitrate compounds). For the oven method, lay the bacon flat on a rimmed baking sheet and bake at 400°F for 15-20 minutes. Drain the fat. For the microwave, layer the bacon with paper towels on a paper plate. Cook for 5 minutes.

2. Meanwhile, heat a cast-iron skillet or heavy saucepan on medium heat. Gently wash the mushrooms and pat them dry. Slice them and add them to the pan, without oil. Cook them, stirring occasionally, until they have released a lot of water and started to turn golden brown. This will concentrate their flavor.

3. Add the olive oil, garlic, bacon, and spinach. Cook until the spinach wilts, about 1 minutes. Reduce heat to medium-low.

4. Turn on the broiler to medium or low. In a medium bowl, beat the eggs together until well combined. Pour them into the skillet and stir gently until the eggs begin to set, about 5 minutes. Place the skillet under the broiler and cook for 5-7 minutes, until the eggs are fully set. Serve hot or cold.

Super Tender Stewed Chicken with Vegetables

Ingredients

2-3 organic, pastured chicken thighs

¼ cup ghee

1 onion

2 cloves garlic

1 small bunch parsley, tied with cooking twine

spices to taste: you can use ginger, and black pepper for a Moroccan flavor; saffron and smoked paprika for a Spanish flavor; or thyme, bay, and rosemary for a French flavor.

¼ tsp salt

2 large carrots

1 zucchini

1 medium potato

Directions

1. Heat the ghee in a large pot. Add the onion, garlic, and spices. Add the chicken thighs and rub to coat with the oil and spice mixture.

2. Cook on the stove top over medium for about 30 minutes, turning occasionally until the chicken is mostly done and has released water.

3. Add 1½ cups of water and cook on low for about 30 minutes.

4. Add the carrots and potatoes and cook for 15 minutes, then add the zucchini. Cook for about 15 more minutes, until the chicken and vegetables are all very tender.

Chilean Chacero Salad

This recipe is based on a delicious Chilean sandwich made with grilled or roast beef, green beans, tomatoes, and cilantro aioli. We've turned it into an equally mouthwatering Whole Food-friendly salad.

Ingredients

½ pound organic 100% grass-fed steak

2 tomatoes

½ pound green beans

2 cloves garlic

1 bag or head heart lettuce, such as Romaine

1 tbsp extra-virgin olive oil

salt and pepper

a few sprigs cilantro

½ cup Homemade Mayonnaise (or Whole30-approved mayo)

Directions

1. Make the aioli. In a blender, mix the cilantro, 1 clove garlic, and mayonnaise until well combined. If you do not have a blender, simply mince the garlic and finely chop the cilantro, and mix them into the mayonnaise.

2. Heat your grill or broiler to medium-high. Toss the green beans with olive oil, salt and pepper, and one clove of minced garlic. Put them in a grill basket or on a doubled-over piece of aluminum foil. Rub the steak with a bit of olive oil and salt and pepper.

3. Grill the steak for about 7 minutes per side, until it is medium rare (or more to your liking). Grill the green beans for about the same amount of time, until they are tender and have a few spots of darker brown.

4. Allow the steak to rest while you prepare the other ingredients. Divide the lettuce between two plates. Slice the tomatoes and arrange them on top of the lettuce. Top with tomatoes with the green beans and finally with the steak. Drizzle the cilantro aioli over the top and serve.

Classic Roast Chicken

Ingredients

1 small roasting chicken, organic and pasture-raised

2 tsp coarse kosher salt

Herbs to taste: grated lemon zest, grated garlic, thyme, rosemary, etc.

2 large carrots

1 medium onion

Directions

1. Wash the chicken and pat it dry with paper towels. Place the chicken on a rack on a baking sheet.

2. Mix together the salt and whatever herbs you are using, and sprinkle the mixture over the chicken. Let it rest, uncovered for at least one and up to 24 hours in the fridge.

3. Preheat the oven to 325 or 450°F. The lower temperature will give you tender flesh and softer skin and require about 1½ hours to cook. The higher temperature will give you crisper, darker skin and firmer meat, and will take 50-60 minutes. Both work!

4. Peel the carrots and chop them into 1-inch pieces. Peel the onion cut into eighths. Scatter the vegetables in the bottom of the roasting pan or skillet.

5. Set the chicken in a roasting pan or a cast-iron skillet. If using a cast-iron skillet, you can preheat it in the oven, which will help ensure even cooking.

6. Roast the chicken until an instant-read thermometer gives an a temperature of 165°F, about 1½ hours for the lower temperature and 50-60 minutes for the higher temperature. A thermometer is the most accurate way to tell if it is done, but you can also cut into a piece and check to see if the juices run clear. When it is nearly done, baste it with the juices that have collected in the bottom of the pan.

7. Remove the chicken from the oven and cover it with aluminum foil. Allow it to rest for 30 minutes, then carve and serve with the roasted carrots on the side.

Stuffed Bell Peppers

Ingredients

2 large bell peppers

1 onion

1 clove garlic

½ tsp cumin

¼ tsp cayenne pepper

pinch salt and black pepper

¼ tsp oregano

½ pound organic grass-fed ground beef

1 small zucchini

1 tomato

1 tbsp extra-virgin olive oil, divided

Directions

1. Finely dice the onion and mince the garlic. Grate the zucchini and the tomato. Cut the top off the peppers. Save the top but scrape out the seeds.

2. Meanwhile, preheat the oven to 400°F. Lightly brush the peppers with olive oil and put them in the oven on a small pan or tray while you work on the filling. This will help the peppers cook fully.

3. Heat a large pan over medium high and add 2 tsp olive oil. Add the onions and garlic and cook until softened. Add the salt and spices.

4. Add the ground beef and continue to cook until fully browned.

5. Add the zucchini and tomato, and cook until most of the water is evaporate and the mixture starts to form a thicker sauce.

6. Take the peppers out of the oven and stand them upright. Fill each of them with half the filling, put the tops of the peppers on, and return them to the oven. Bake for 20-30 minutes, until the peppers have softened.

Squash Stir-Fry

Ingredients

1 medium butternut squash

2 cups mushrooms 1-2 tbsp ghee

1 onion

Salt and black pepper

2 cloves garlic

¼ chili powder

1-inch piece fresh ginger

1 tbsp toasted sesame oil

1 tbsp apple cider vinegar

Directions

1. Peel and cube the butternut squash. Dice the onion. Mince the garlic. Rinse and slice the mushrooms. Peel and grate the ginger.

1. Place it in a large microwave-safe bowl and cook for 8 minutes on high, until somewhat tender.

2. Meanwhile, heat a large frying pan over medium heat. Add all the mushrooms, and cook for 6-7 minutes. This allows some of their water to evaporate, developing and concentrating the flavor.

3. Add the ghee and the onions, and increase the heat. Cook for 2 minutes, then add the garlic, ginger, and chili. Cook just until they are fragrant, and add the squash.

4. Cook until the squash starts to show golden-brown edges and is tender inside. Add the vinegar and sesame oil and cook for 1 more minute. Serve.

Creamy Spiced Sweet Potato Soup

Ingredients

2 medium sweet potatoes

½ small onion

2 tbsp ghee

¼ chili powder

½-inch piece fresh ginger, peeled and grated

¼ tsp cinnamon

1/8 tsp cloves

¼ tsp allspice

½ cup cashews, soaked overnight

3 cups vegetable or chicken broth

Directions

1. The night before you plan to make the soup, cover the cashews with water and let them soak overnight in the fridge.

2. Peel the sweet potatoes and chop them into small cubes. Put them in a large microwave-safe bowl and microwave on high for 7 minutes, or until they are mostly cooked. This step is optional – you can cook them on the stovetop in the broth – but it will greatly speed up the process.

3. Meanwhile, heat the ghee in a medium pot. Add the onion and spices, and cook, stirring frequently, until the onion is softened and translucent.

4. Add the broth, sweet potatoes, and cashews, and cook until the sweet potatoes are completely soft. Add more broth or water as needed.

5. Allow the soup to cool slightly, then transfer to a blender or food processor and blend until very smooth. You can add more liquid in this step too if desired. Reheat and serve.

Broiled Spring Vegetables with Poached Eggs

Ingredients

½ pound asparagus

4 shallots

¼ pound sugar snap peas

1 tbsp extra-virgin olive oil

salt and pepper

½ lemon

4 eggs

2 tbsp white vinegar

Directions

1. Peel and thinly slice the shallots. Wash and trim the asparagus. Rinse the sugar snap peas. Set the broiler to high and position the rack about 6 inches below the heat source.

2. Toss all the vegetables with olive oil, salt, and pepper, and spread them on a flat pan. Put them in the broiler and cook for 7-8 minutes, checking and shaking the pan occasionally, until the shallots are translucent and the peas and asparagus are bright green with edges just slightly blackened.

3. Meanwhile, poach the eggs. Bring a sauce pan with 3 inches of water to a low simmer and add the vinegar. Crack the eggs into small bowl and very

gently lower and tilt the eggs into the water. Cook for 3-4 minutes..

4. Divide the vegetables between two plates and squeeze some lemon juice over them. Once the eggs are done, carefully scoop them out of the water with a slotted spoon. Allow them to drain for a moment, then place them on top of the vegetables. Salt and pepper to taste and serve.

Meaty Salsa Salad

Ingredients

1 medium sized onion, chopped

2 Tablespoons of red chili powder

3 cups of cherry tomatoes, cut into halves

½ teaspoon of cayenne pepper

¼ cup of coconut sour cream,

2 Romaine hearts, chopped

½ cup of homemade vinaigrette

2 cloves of garlic, minced

1 Tablespoon of fresh lime juice

1 lb of lean ground beef

2 teaspoons of garlic powder

½ cup of chopped fresh cilantro, to garnish

2 teaspoons of ground cumin

Kosher salt to taste

Freshly grounded black pepper to taste

Directions

1. Combine the chili powder, kosher salt, ground cumin, garlic powder, black pepper and cayenne pepper in a bowl. Mix all the spices well then set aside.

2. Take a non-stick skillet and heat it over medium flame.

3. Put the meat in it and cook until it is browned.

4. When the meat is brown, add the minced garlic and onion to it.

5. Cook and stir until the onion loses its colour and becomes translucent.

6. Now put the spice mixture in it and mix well.

7. Cook for about three more minutes, while stirring continuously.

8. Now take another mixing bowl and put the coconut sour cream in it. Then add in it the lime juice and vinaigrette. Mix well.

9. Spread the chopped lettuce on a serving platter.

10. Place the meat over the lettuce followed by the cream-salsa mixture.

11. Garnish with fresh cilantro and tomatoes.

12. Enjoy!

Pork Delight

Ingredients

1 Tablespoon of fresh lime juice

2 onions, thinly sliced

Half cup of fresh cilantro, finely chopped

1 red bell peppers, thinly sliced

2 Tablespoons of extra virgin olive oil

2 Tablespoons of olive oil, divided

1 lb of pork tenderloin, thinly sliced

4 clove of garlic cloves, finely diced

1 Tablespoon of finely chopped ginger

Directions

1. Take a large mixing bowl and combine the ginger, garlic, extra virgin olive oil and chopped cilantro in it. Mix well.

2. Place the pork slices in this bowl. Flip to coat all the sides of the meat with this mixture. Set aside to marinade for about an hour.

3. After an hour, take a non-stick pan, put it over medium high flame and heat half of the olive oil in it.

4. Brown the marinated pork strips in it. When the pork is well done, turn off the flame.

5. Take another non-stick pan, put it over medium high flame and heat the remaining olive oil in it.

6. Put the onions in this pan.

7. Cook till the onions lose their colour and become translucent.

8. Stir in the chopped bell pepper.

9. Cook and stir for about five more minutes.

10. Stir in the pork slices. Cook and stir for two more minutes.

11. Add the fresh lime juice in this pan. Cook for one more minute, then dish out.

12. Enjoy!

Grilled Pork Chops with Veggies

Ingredients

3 cloves of garlic, crushed and divided

4 (¾ inch thick) pork chops, bone-in and trimmed

1 teaspoon of extra virgin olive oil, divided

4 teaspoons of chili powder, divided

2 Tablespoons of ghee

3 Tablespoons of white vinegar

6 cups of Napa cabbage, thinly sliced

4 scallions, thinly sliced

4 radishes, chopped into small strips

½ teaspoon of sea salt

Directions

1. Firstly, grease the grill and then preheat the griller to medium heat.

2. Now combine the ghee, one crushed clove, half of the chili powder and white vinegar in a large bowl. Whisk well.

3. Add the cabbage, radishes and scallions to the bowl. Stir to mix. Set aside.

4. Now combine remaining garlic, the remaining chili powder and salt in another mixing bowl. Mix well

then add olive oil to it. Mix well. Now coat the chops in this mixture.

5. Make sure both sides of the chops are thoroughly coated in it.

6. Now grill the chops. Grill on one side for five minutes, flip over and then grill another side for five minutes, until the chops are done.

7. Place the grilled chops in a serving platter.

8. Serve with the Napa cabbage veggie mixture.

9. Enjoy!

Negative Calorie Burger

Ingredients

¾ kg lean minced beef or chicken

¼ tsp. sea salt

½ tsp. all-spice

½ tsp. cayenne pepper, optional

½ tsp. ground black pepper

1 tbsp. coconut oil

Directions

1. Mix all the ingredients together and create six patties.

2. Place a skillet over medium heat and pour the oil when hot.

3. Cook the burgers to desired doneness.

4. Enjoy!

Classic Beef Stew

Ingredients

1 kg lean beef, cubed

1 large red onion

2 cloves garlic, minced

2 small carrots

3 cups canned tomatoes

1 tsp. basil

1 tsp. oregano

3 cups beef stock

1/2 cup white vinegar

1 tsp. salt

1 tbsp. olive oil

3 potatoes, peeled and diced

Directions

1. In a large pot, pour the oil and allow to heat then add the beef. Stir until evenly browned. Add the onion and garlic until soft. Mix for about 2 minutes then add the carrots.

2. Add all the other ingredients cover and cook on very low heat for about 2 hours until the beef is tender.

3. Enjoy!

Chicken topped with Mango Salsa

Ingredients:

1 lb. boneless chicken breast

1/4 cup lime juice

2 Tbsp. avocado oil

1 handful fresh cilantro

1/2 tsp. chilli powder

salt and pepper to taste

Mango salsa ingredients:

1 tomato, diced

1 mango, diced

3 Tbsp. lime juice

1 avocado, diced

1/2 Tbsp. red wine vinegar

1/4 cup cilantro, diced

Directions

1. Add all of the cilantro lime chicken ingredients in together and whisk until mixed. Add chicken and marinade in a large ziplock bag.

2. Let chicken marinade for at least 15 minutes.

3. Preheat grill to medium heat and place chicken on the grill and grill each side for around 5 minutes, until chicken is no longer pink.

4. To make the mango salsa add all of the salsa ingredients together and gently toss to mix. Top the cilantro lime chicken with mango salsa and enjoy.

Grilled Chicken Over Squash Spaghetti

Ingredients:

2-3 cups spiralized squash

1 cup grilled chicken, chopped or shredded

1 avocado, pitted

2 cloves garlic, crushed

2 tbsp. coconut milk

2 tbsp. olive oil

2 tbsp. lemon juice

¼ cup sun-dried tomatoes packed in oil

Handful of fresh basil

Kosher salt and freshly ground pepper to taste

Directions:

1. Combine avocado, garlic, coconut milk, lemon juice, basil, salt and pepper in a food processor and pulse until they become smooth.

2. Pour a bit of olive oil in a medium skillet over medium heat and sauté the squash spaghetti until desired tenderness is achieved for about 8 minutes.

3. Stir in the avocado sauce, tomatoes and chicken until they are well combined. Cook until heated through. Add some water if the sauce is too thick. Turn off the heat and garnish with chopped basil.

4. Serve immediately and enjoy!

Spicy Chicken Cilantro Wraps

Ingredients

3 cups cooked and shredded chicken

Juice of 1 lime

3 green onions, sliced

¼ cup cilantro, chopped

¼ teaspoon chili powder

¼ teaspoon cumin

¼ teaspoon garlic powder

¼ teaspoon of cayenne pepper

Sea salt and pepper to taste

½ avocado, mashed

Leaf lettuce for serving

Directions

1. Mix together all ingredients except the leaf lettuce in a bowl until well combined.

2. Wrap the mixture in lettuce leaves or, alternatively, stuff inside a tomato or avocado.

3. Enjoy!

Arugula Salmon Salad

Ingredients:

1 cup of arugula

2 Tbsp. of chopped walnuts

1 can of wild caught salmon

1 pear, thinly sliced

Dressing:

2 Tbsp. of olive oil

1 Tbsp. French mustard

1/2 tsp sea salt

Directions

1. -Start by making the dressing, by whisking together the olive oil with the French mustard, and sea salt.

2. -Assemble the salad with the arugula as the base, and top with sliced pears, chopped walnuts, and the wild caught salmon.

3. -Drizzle with the homemade dressing.

Gazpacho & Guacamole

Ingredients:

<u>For the gazpacho</u>

4 large, vine-ripened tomatoes

1 cucumber, chopped

1 zucchini. chopped

4 mini-sweet peppers, chopped

1 small red onion, finely chopped

1 jalapeno, deseeded and finely chopped

2 garlic cloves, minced

¼ cup olive oil

3 cups vegetable, chicken, or beef broth

2 tablespoons red wine vinegar

Coarse sea salt

Freshly ground pepper

<u>For the guacamole</u>

1 Haas avocado, diced

¼ cup diced red onion

1 clove of garlic, minced

juice of 1 lime

Directions

1. Preheat oven to 450 degrees Fahrenheit.

2. Quarter the tomatoes and place on a baking sheet. Drizzle with olive oil and sprinkle with salt and pepper. Bake in oven for 30-35 minutes, until slightly browned. Remove and allow to cool.

3. In a food processor or high speed blender, pulse the chopped vegetables together and place in a large bowl. Add the tomatoes to the food processor and blender and blend until smooth. Add the vegetable mixture.

4. Stir in the olive oil, broth, and red wine vinegar. Cover and chill for at least 2 hours.

5. For the guacamole, simply mix all ingredients in a bowl, mashing the avocado with a fork.

6. Serve the gazpacho with a dollop of guacamole on top and enjoy!

Salmon Avocado Boats

Serves: 2

Serving Size: 2 avocado halves

Ingredients

2 ripe avocados

4 oz. wild caught smoked salmon

2 green onions, thinly sliced

2 tablespoons olive oil

Juice of one lemon

Sea salt and pepper to taste

Directions

1. Cut the avocados in half lengthwise and remove the seed.

2. In a small food processor or magic bullet, pulse the salmon with the olive oil and lemon juice.

3. Stir in the sliced green onions and season with salt and pepper.

4. Divide the mixture evenly between the avocado halves.

5. Serve immediately.

Roasted Red Pepper and Egg Bake

Serves: 4

Ingredients

4 red bell peppers, halved lengthwise and seeded

5 large eggs

½ cup coconut milk

3 green onions, sliced

½ cup frozen spinach, thawed and drained

4 slices bacon, cooked and crumbled

Sea salt and pepper to taste

Directions

1. Preheat oven to 350 degrees Fahrenheit.

2. In a medium bowl, whisk the eggs and coconut milk together. Add the green onion, spinach, and bacon. Mix until well combined and season with salt and pepper.

3. Place the bell pepper halves in a lightly greased baking dish.

4. Divide the egg mixture between the peppers. Cover with foil and cook for 45 minutes, until the eggs are set.

5. Serve immediately.

Ham and Cauliflower Fritters

Serves: 4

Serving Size: 3-4 fritters

Ingredients

1 head cauliflower

3 large eggs

1 ½ cup diced ham

1 clove garlic, minced

Sea salt and pepper to taste

Coconut oil for frying

Directions

1. Chop the cauliflower into ½" pieces and steam for 10-15 minutes, until soft. Drain well and mash with a fork or potato masher, pressing to release as much liquid as possible.

2. Transfer the cauliflower to a large bowl. Add the eggs, ham, and garlic. Season with salt and pepper.

3. Heat a large skillet over medium heat and about a tablespoon of coconut oil.

4. Form the cauliflower mixture into flat patties, using about 2-3 tablespoons per patty.

5. Once the oil is hot, add a few patties and cook for 3-5 minutes per side.

6. Remove to a paper towel lined plate and repeat with the remaining patties.

7. Serve hot.

One serving of cauliflower contains 77% of your daily recommended amount vitamin C. It's also a good source of fiber, potassium, and protein, believe it or not!

Chicken and Mushroom Crepes

Serves: 4

Serving Size: 1 crepe

Ingredients

4 large eggs

2 cups coconut milk

1 cup mushrooms, thinly sliced

1 yellow onion, thinly sliced

2 boneless, skinless chicken breasts, cut into ½" pieces

4 slices bacon, cooked and chopped

Sea salt and pepper to taste

Olive oil for the pan

Directions

1. Whisk the eggs together with about a tablespoon of coconut milk and season with salt and pepper.

2. Heat a small pan over medium heat and add a bit of olive oil.

3. Pour approximately ½ cup of the egg mixture into the pan and swirl to evenly coat the pan.

4. Once the eggs have set, flip and cook for about 1 minute. Transfer to a paper towel lined plate and repeat 3 times with the remaining egg mixture.

5. In a large pan, sauté the chicken, onions, and mushrooms until the chicken is cooked through. Season with salt and pepper.

6. Stir in half of the bacon and the remaining coconut milk. Cook about 3-4 minutes, until slightly thickened.

7. Divide the chicken mixture between the 4 egg crepes, fold, and top with remaining bacon.

8. Serve and enjoy!

For thousands of years, mushrooms have been celebrated as a powerful source for nutrients. They are a good source of B vitamins, which play an important role in the nervous system. They also contain high amounts of selenium, a mineral that is important to the immune system.

Cream of Chicken Soup

Serves: 4

Serving Size: 8 oz.

Ingredients

4 cups homemade beef or chicken broth

2 boneless, skinless chicken breasts, chopped into ½" pieces

2 shallots, diced

1 yellow onion, diced

6-8 cloves garlic, minced

2 cups coconut milk (canned)

2 tablespoons coconut aminos

¼ cup coconut oil

3 teaspoons thyme

1 teaspoon sea salt

1 teaspoon black pepper

½ cup flat leaf parsley, chopped (to garnish)

Directions

1. In a large stock pot over medium-high heat, sauté the onions, shallots, and garlic in the coconut oil until translucent.

2. Add the chicken and continue sautéing until the chicken is cooked through.

3. Season with the thyme, salt, and pepper.

4. Stir in the broth and coconut aminos. Bring to a simmer. Reduce heat to low and cook for 30-35 minutes.

5. Add the coconut milk and cook for an additional 5 minutes. Remove from heat.

6. Using an immersion blender, or working in small batches with a regular blender, puree the soup until smooth and creamy.

7. Top with chopped parsley and serve!

Homemade broth has anti-inflammatory and gut healing properties as well as being high in proteins, healthy fats, and minerals.

Beef Stuffed Zucchini Boats

Serves: 2

Serving Size: 2 boats

Ingredients

1-pound ground beef

2 ½ cups cauliflower "rice"

4 large zucchini

3 tablespoons Dijon mustard

Sea salt and pepper to taste

¼ teaspoon garlic salt

Directions

1. Preheat oven to 350 degrees Fahrenheit.

2. Trim the ends off the zucchini and cut in half lengthwise. Using a small spoon, scoop out the seeds and core of the zucchini. Dice and reserve for later use.

3. In a large skillet, brown the ground beef until mostly cooked. Add the cauliflower "rice" (this can be made by pulsing the cauliflower florets in your food processor) and zucchini core. Cook for 2-3 minutes. Add the Dijon mustard and season with salt, pepper, and garlic salt. Cook for 1-2 minutes until heated through.

4. Season the zucchini boats with salt and pepper and fill with the beef mixture.

5. Place on a baking sheet, cover with foil, and bake for 20 minutes.

6. Remove foil and bake an additional 10 minutes, until golden brown.

7. Serve and enjoy!

Zucchini is an excellent source of dietary fiber and contains high amounts of potassium, an important electrolyte that can help to reduce blood pressure.

Shrimp Ceviche

Serves: 3

Serving Size: 1 cup

Ingredients

2 pounds raw shrimp

1 large tomato, diced

2 cloves garlic, minced

1 jalapeno, seeded and diced

½ avocado, diced

Juice of 1 orange

Juice of 2 lemons

Juice of 2 limes

¼ cup cilantro, chopped

Sea salt and pepper

Directions

1. Peel and devein the shrimp. Chop into small pieces.

2. Mix the shrimp with the tomato, garlic, jalapeno, and avocado.

3. Squeeze the citrus juice on top and mix well. There should be enough juice to completely cover the shrimp.

4. Refrigerate at least 6 hours or until the shrimp has turned from translucent to opaque.

5. Season with salt and pepper and top with chopped cilantro.

A four ounce serving of shrimp supplies 23.7 grams of protein. Combine that with the healthy dose of vitamin C from the citrus in this recipe and you've got a lunch that's as tasty as it is nutritional.

Mayo Free Chicken Salad

Serves: 4

Serving Size: 1 cup

Ingredients

4 cups cooked chicken, chopped

2 cups zucchini, peeled and diced

1/3 cup coconut cream

1 teaspoon garlic powder

½ cup fresh cilantro

Juice of ½ a lemon

Sea salt to taste

Directions

1. Add all ingredients except the chicken to a food processor or magic bullet.

2. Process until combined. If too thick, add a bit more lemon juice.

3. Place the chopped chicken in a bowl and top with the sauce.

4. Stir until the chicken is thoroughly coated.

5. Serve atop a bed of salad greens and enjoy!

Skinny vegetable-beef soup

Ingredients

6 carrots, chopped

1 red pepper, chopped

1 green pepper, chopped

4 cups thickly sliced mushrooms

10 celery stalks with leaves on, chopped

1 small head of garlic, finely chopped

4 onions, chopped

4 cups chopped cabbage

2 cups chopped broccoli

1 small bunch parsley

1 small bunch cilantro, chopped

1 cup frozen spinach

1 cup canned artichokes, rinsed and drained

1 can asparagus, rinsed and drained

2 cans diced tomatoes with basil

2 cans green beans, rinsed and drained

2 cans tomatoes with green chili

450g lean ground beef

Freshly cracked black pepper to taste

1 tbsp. Italian seasoning

1 tbsp. dried basil

½ tbsp. red pepper flakes

8 cups low sodium beef broth

You are going to need:

An extra-large soup pot

Directions

1. Fill your soup pot halfway up with the broth and add all the chopped veggies, herbs and spices. Bring to a boil over high heat then lower the heat and simmer.
2. Meanwhile, fry your ground beef until browned then add to the soup pot.
3. Simmer for 1 hour until all the veggies are tender and add some more broth if your soup boils down.
4. Serve hot.
5. Enjoy!

Yummy cauliflower and roasted asparagus soup

Ingredients

8 cups cauliflower florets

450g asparagus stalks, spears trimmed

4 cups homemade vegetable broth

1 tsp minced garlic

1 onion, minced

A pinch of cayenne pepper

Freshly ground pepper to taste

Sea salt to taste

Directions

1. Start by setting your oven to 400F.
2. Arrange the asparagus and cauliflower florets on a baking sheet and bake for about 20 minutes until cauliflower starts turning golden and the asparagus is fork tender.
3. Combine the roasted veggies, garlic and onion with the broth in a large soup pot and cook on low heat for 15 minutes. Use an immersion blender to puree the soup to desired consistency.
4. Season your soup and cook for 1 more minute.
5. Serve in soup bowls.
6. Enjoy!

Minty cucumber salad

Ingredients

1 cucumber, very thinly sliced using a mandolin

2 carrots, thinly sliced

½ a Vidalia onion, thinly sliced

1/3 cup white vinegar

3 packets stevia (this is a zero calorie natural sweetener)

Freshly squeezed juice of 1 lime

2 tbsp. fresh mint, chopped

1/3 cup water

Sea salt to taste

Freshly ground pepper to taste

Directions

1. Sprinkle the sliced cucumbers with sea salt and let it sit for 20 minutes then rinse out the salt and squeeze out the excess water.
2. Make the salad dressing and marinate the cucumber, carrots and onions and refrigerate for 2 hours.
3. Toss the salad ingredients with thee chopped mint in a salad bowl.
4. Enjoy!

Berries and greens salad with poppy seed dressing

Ingredients

3cups arugula leaves, roughly torn

3 cups watercress leaves

3 cups strawberries, sliced

2 tsp. poppy seeds

¼ cup freshly squeezed orange juice

½ tsp freshly grated orange rind

Directions

1. Combine the greens with the strawberries in a salad bowl then set aside.
2. Whisk the orange juice, orange rind and poppy seeds in a separate bowl then pour over the berry-greens mixture.
3. Toss well to combine and serve immediately or chill in the fridge until you are ready to serve.
4. Enjoy!

Juicy lime shrimp salad

Ingredients

225g large shrimp, peeled, deveined and cleaned

Bibb lettuce leaves

1 tbsp. chopped red pepper

1 scallion, chopped (both the green and white parts)

1 ½ tbsp. freshly squeezed lime juice

½ tsp extra virgin olive oil

½ tbsp. hoisin sauce

¼ tsp minced garlic

1 tbsp. freshly chopped cilantro

A pinch if white pepper

Directions

1. Combine the hoisin sauce, lime juice, white pepper, cilantro, olive oil, garlic, scallions and white pepper. Whisk well to combine then set aside.
2. Heat a tablespoon of this mixture in a non-stick pan over medium heat then add the shrimp. Cook for about 3 minutes tossing frequently until the shrimp turns opaque.

3. Now pour the shrimp mixture into the lime juice mixture and toss in the red pepper. Cover the bowl using cling wrap and refrigerate for 30 minutes, tossing every 10 minutes or so.
4. Line serving plates with the Bibb lettuce leaves and spoon the salad over the lettuce. Drizzle a little of the marinade on top.
5. Enjoy!

Mains Recipes

Herbed chicken and veggie stir-fry

Ingredients

4 pcs broiled chicken breast

1 small bunch asparagus, ends trimmed and cut into bite size pieces

4 fresh garlic cloves

1 tbsp. Canola oil

1 red onion, sliced

1 small bunch celery, cut into bite size pieces

8 cherry tomatoes, cut in quarters

1 cup freshly chopped basil leaves

A dash of flaxseed oil

A dash of low-sodium soy sauce

Directions

1. Boil the chicken breasts until lightly browned and completely cooked through then set aside.
2. Heat the canola and flaxseed oil in a large wok and sauté the whole garlic cloves until soft. Add in the sliced onions, tomatoes, celery and asparagus into the garlic-flavored oil.
3. Shred the boiled chicken and add it to the veggies. Add the basil leaves and stir everything together for about 3-5 minutes.
4. Add the soy sauce and cook for one more minute.
5. Serve piping hot and crisp, you want the veggies to have a firm bite to them.
6. Enjoy!

Citrusy baked salmon with bulgur and asparagus

Ingredients

600g skinless salmon fillet, divided into 4 pieces

450g asparagus, trimmed1 ½ cups low sodium chicken or veggie broth

1 cup bulgur

2 tbsp. freshly chopped dill

1 lemon, thinly sliced

¼ tsp Kosher salt or to taste

¼ tsp Freshly ground black pepper or to taste

Extra virgin olive oil, for serving

Directions

1. Start by setting your oven to 375F.
2. Combine the bulgur and broth in a shallow baking dish and season with the salt and pepper.
3. Gently arrange the asparagus on top on a single layer. Place the salmon fillets on top and season with salt and pepper then top with the lemon slices.
4. Use foil to tightly cover the dish and bake for 30 minutes or until salmon is cooked through and the asparagus and bulgur are tender.
5. Divide among four plates and top with chopped dill and drizzle with olive oil.
6. Enjoy!

Wild Grilled Salmon

Ingredients

2 cloves of garlic, minced

2 (1 ½ lbs. each) fillets of wild salmon fillet

2 tomatoes, thinly sliced

2 cups of fresh basil, finely chopped

Olive oil cooking spray

Half teaspoons of freshly ground black pepper

2 Tablespoons of olive oil

2 teaspoons of kosher salt

Directions

1. Set the grill to preheat at medium.

2. Take aluminum foil, cut two large pieces of it and place it over another to make double layer of the foil. Now coat this foil with cooking spray.

3. Place both the fillets on the prepared aluminum foil. Make sure you put them skin side down and both the fillets should be placed apart each other. Do not overlap.

4. Now take a small bowl and combine the salt, minced garlic and oil in it. Mix well. Brush it over the salmon fillets.

5. Place the tomatoes slices on top of the fillets and spread the fresh basil over the tomatoes.

6. Put in the preheated griller and grill for about 15 minutes, until the fish flakes.

7. Place the grilled fish on a serving plate.

8. Serve it hot! Enjoy!

Mexican Beef Stuffed Peppers

Ingredients

1 teaspoon of garlic powder

Half cup of fresh cilantro, chopped

4 ounces black olives, chopped into slices

4 yellow bell peppers, seeds removed and cut into halves

1 lb of lean ground beef

10 ounces tomatoes with green chilies (canned)

6 ounces tomato paste

3 ripe avocados, pitted and peeled

1 large onion, finely chopped

Olive oil cooking spray

Homemade seasoning for marinade

Directions

1. Marinate the meat with the homemade seasoning. Set aside for a while.

2. Preheat the oven to 300 degrees Fahrenheit.

3. Take a baking dish and grease it with cooking spray.

4. Heat a non-stick skillet and place the marinated beef in it.

5. Cook until the beef is browned.

6. When the meat is done, add cilantro and onions to it.

7. Cook and stir for five minutes.

8. Take one half of the half-cut peppers and finely chop them.

9. Mix the chopped peppers to the beef-onion mixture.

10. Stir in the olives, tomato paste and tomatoes with green chilies. Mix well.

11. Put all the remaining peppers, open side up, in the prepared baking dish.

12. Stuff each open half of the pepper with equal portions of the beef mixture.

13. Bake for about half an hour.

14. In the meantime, put the avocados in a bowl along with the garlic powder.

15. Using a potato masher or two forks, mash the avocados and then stir to mix with the garlic powder.

16. Once the peppers in the oven are done, set them in a serving dish.

17. Garnish each pepper with equal amount of the avocado mixture.

18. Serve it hot. Enjoy!

Greek Roast Lamb

The Whole30 is a great opportunity to try meats you might not cook with as often. Lamb is a rich, flavorful meat that goes well with vegetables and strong spices. This recipe serves 6-8.

Ingredients

1 leg of organic, grass-fed lamb (4-5 pounds)

8 cloves garlic

10 sprigs oregano

¼ cup extra-virgin olive oil

1 tsp salt

2 pounds potatoes

1 large onion

2 lemons

Directions

1. Preheat the oven to 350°F. Peel the potatoes and cut them into eighths. Cut the onion into eighths and quarter the lemons. Scatter them all in the bottom of a large roasting pan.

2. Take the garlic, oregano, salt, and oil and pound them together into a paste. You can use a mortar and pestle, or mince the garlic and oregano and then stir it into the oil and salt.

3. Set the leg of lamb in the roasting pan on top of the vegetables. Using a sharp knife, cut about 30 small slits in the meat. Rub the spice mixture into the leg of lamb, working as much as possible into the slits.

4. Pour one cup of water into the pan and put it in the oven. Roast the lamb for 1½-2 hours for medium rare, turning the leg over about halfway through. Remove the lamb from the oven, cover with foil, and allow to rest for 30 minutes before carving and serving.

Curried Vegetables with Cauliflower 'Rice'

Ingredients

1 head cauliflower

1 medium potato

3 large carrots

1 green bell pepper

2 cups spinach (You can substitute whatever vegetables you like)

2 tsp extra-virgin olive oil

2 cloves garlic

1 tsp turmeric

1 tsp paprika

½ tsp cayenne pepper

½ tsp cumin

½ tsp coriander (You can substitute 2-3 tsp curry powder for the spices)

½ can coconut milk

¼ cup golden raisins

¼ cup cashews

Directions

1. Peel the potato and carrots and chop them into ½-inch pieces. Dice the pepper. Mince the garlic. Chop the cauliflower into a few large chunks.

2. Heat the oil over medium in a large pan. Add the garlic and all the spices and cook for 2 minutes, until they are fragrant. Add the potato, carrots, and peppers and cook for 6-7 minutes, or until the potatoes and carrots start to soften.

3. Meanwhile, heat 1 inch of water in a medium pot. Add the cauliflower pieces, cover, and steam for 3-4 minutes, until the cauliflower is softened but still quite firm. Transfer the cauliflower to a food processor and pulse a few times until the cauliflower is completely broken up into rice-size pieces.

4. Add the spinach to the other vegetables and stir until it wilts. Add the coconut milk, golden raisins, and cashews. Simmer the curry until the vegetables are tender, about 10 minutes.

5. Divide the cauliflower between two plates. Once the curry is done, spoon it over the cauliflower and serve.

Baked Beef with Mushroom and Squash

Ingredients

¼ cup of fresh basil, chopped

¼ cup of water

1 ½ lbs of lean ground beef

¼ cup of fresh thyme, chopped

1 spaghetti squash, seeded and halved

1 medium white onion, chopped

¼ cup of fresh oregano, chopped

1 Tablespoon of red pepper flakes

1 red bell pepper, chopped

1 cup of mushrooms, sliced

2 ¾ cups of crushed tomatoes

1 medium sized zucchini, diced

1 green bell pepper, chopped

1 Tablespoon of extra virgin olive oil

Directions

1. Preheat the oven to 400 degrees Fahrenheit.

2. Take a baking dish and pour the water in it.

3. Place the squash halves in the water in the baking dish.

4. Put this dish in the oven for about 35 minutes, until the squash is soft enough to grate.

5. In the meantime, heat a non-stick pan over medium high flame.

6. Put the beef and onion in the pan.

7. Cook and stir until the beef is browned and slightly crumbled.

8. When the beef is done, turn off the flame.

9. Now take another non-stick pan, put the oil in it and heat it over medium flame.

10. Put the zucchini, mushrooms, green bell pepper and red bell peppers in the oil.

11. Cook and stir until all the vegetables are slightly soft but crispy.

12. Then add the fresh basil, oregano, crushed tomatoes and thyme in it.

13. Simmer over medium heat for about ten minutes.

14. Now put the beef mixture in it. Mix well.

15. Reduce the heat of the stove to low.

16. Cook while stirring occasionally for about five minutes, then set aside.

17. When the squash is soft, carefully shred or coarsely mash it with the help of two forks.

18. Put this in the cooked beef mixture. Stir to mix.

19. Enjoy!

Tuna Burgers

Ingredients

1 Tablespoon of grated ginger root

9 ½ ounces tuna (canned and drained)

Half cup of almond meal

About 1 Tablespoon of olive oil, for frying

¼ cup of fresh cilantro, chopped

2 Tablespoons of fresh lemon juice

2 Tablespoons of Extra Virgin Olive Oil

3 pastured eggs

Kosher salt to taste

Ground black pepper to taste

Directions

1. Except for the olive oil, combine all the other ingredients in a large bowl. Mix well.

2. Now make four equal portions of the mixture and form a burger from each portion.

3. Heat the olive oil over medium flame in a non-stick skillet.

4. When the oil is hot, fry your burger patties. Fry each side for about five minutes, until the patty is brown and crispy.

5. Serve it as it is or you can also sandwich it between burger buns.

Spicy Beef Roast

Ingredients

29 ounces diced tomatoes

Half teaspoon of red pepper flakes

1 teaspoon of ground ginger

Half teaspoon of ground black pepper

1 teaspoon of sea salt

2 lbs of beef roast, chopped into one-inch chunks

1 teaspoon of ground cinnamon

2 Tablespoons of extra virgin olive oil (substitute: coconut oil)

1 teaspoon of ground turmeric

1 teaspoon of ground cumin

2 teaspoons of paprika

1 medium yellow onion, chopped

5 cloves of garlic, crushed

2 lbs of butternut squash, peeled and chopped into one-inch

Half cup of fresh cilantro, chopped

Directions

1. Except for the last two ingredients (i.e. butternut squash and cilantro), put all the ingredients in a crock pot. Mix well.

2. Cover the crock pot and cook on low flame for about six hours, until the meat is soft.

3. When the meat is tender, add the squash cubes to the crock pot.

4. Again, cover the crock pot and cook on low flame for one hour and 30 minutes, until the squash is tender.

5. Dish out and garnish with fresh cilantro.

6. Enjoy!

Wholesome Pizza

Ingredients

1 Tablespoon of kosher salt

1 teaspoon of red pepper flakes

3 ½ oz. chicken or pork or any other meat, cooked and sliced

1 teaspoon of garlic salt

1 cup of almond cheese, divided

1 cup of tomato sauce

2 lbs of lean ground beef

1 teaspoon of ground black pepper

2 free range eggs

1 teaspoon of caraway seeds

1 teaspoon of dried oregano

Olive oil cooking spray

Directions

1. Preheat the oven to 450 degrees Fahrenheit.

2. Take a pizza pan and grease it with cooking spray.

3. In a small mixing bowl, combine the kosher salt, oregano, garlic salt, ground black pepper, caraway seeds and red pepper flakes. Stir to mix well then set aside.

4. In another mixing bowl, mix the ground beef and eggs.

5. Stir in half of the almond cheese and the spice mixture.

6. Put this beef-cheese mixture into the prepared pizza pan and press it lightly to make an even base.

7. Put it in the preheated oven and bake for about ten minutes, until the meat loses its pinkness.

8. Carefully, take out the pizza pan and then heat up the oven's broiler.

9. Out of the remaining cheese, spread one-third of it over the beef base in the pizza pan.

10. Then spread the tomato sauce over it, followed by another one-third of the cheese.

11. Spread the chicken slices, and finally the remaining cheese.

12. Put it in the broiler for about five minutes, until the cheese is melted and lightly browned on the top.

13. Slice the pizza and serve immediately.

14. Enjoy!

Asian Style Curry

INGREDIENTS

1 ½ pounds boneless, skinless chicken breasts

2 carrots, diced

½ head green cabbage, shredded

3 cups mushrooms, sliced

1 can coconut milk

½ cup chicken stock

1 tablespoon Thai red curry paste

1-2 tablespoons coconut aminos (optional)

1-2 tablespoons fish sauce

½ cup cilantro, roughly chopped

Directions

1. In a large stockpot, combine the coconut milk with the curry paste and bring to a simmer.

2. In the meantime, cut the chicken into 1" pieces.

3. Add the chicken, carrots, chicken broth, fish sauce, and coconut aminos to the coconut milk. Mix well and simmer for 10 minutes.

4. Add the cabbage and mushrooms and cook for 3-5 minutes.

5. Divide into bowls, top with cilantro, and enjoy!

Serves: 4

Thai Red Curry

INGREDIENTS

1 ½ pounds boneless, skinless chicken breasts

2 carrots, diced

½ head green cabbage, shredded

3 cups mushrooms, sliced

1 can coconut milk

½ cup chicken stock

1 tablespoon Thai red curry paste

1-2 tablespoons coconut aminos

1-2 tablespoons fish sauce

½ cup cilantro, roughly chopped

Directions

1. In a large stockpot, combine the coconut milk with the curry paste and bring to a simmer.

2. In the meantime, cut the chicken into 1" pieces.

3. Add the chicken, carrots, chicken broth, fish sauce, and coconut aminos to the coconut milk. Mix well and simmer for 10 minutes.

4. Add the cabbage and mushrooms and cook for 3-5 minutes.

5. Divide into bowls, top with cilantro, and enjoy!

Serves: 4

Fish sauce is an intensely flavored sauce most often made of anchovies, salt, and water. It can be found in the Asian section of most grocery stores, but if unavailable, Worcestershire sauce can be substituted.

Southwestern Meatloaf

INGREDIENTS

1 ½ pounds grass-fed ground beef

1 egg, whisked

1 green pepper, diced

1 red pepper, diced

1 red onion, diced

2 cloves garlic, minced

1 tablespoon chili powder

1 teaspoon smoked paprika

1 teaspoon cumin

 Sea salt and pepper to taste

1 tablespoon olive oil

Directions

1. Preheat oven to 400 degrees Fahrenheit.

2. Heat a large skillet over medium-high heat. Add the olive oil to the pan and sauté the peppers and onion until softened. Remove from heat.

3. Add the ground beef, egg, and spices to a large bowl. Mix well with hands.

4. Transfer the mixture into a loaf pan and cook for 40-45 minutes.

5. Allow to cool for 10-15 minutes before slicing.

6. Serve and enjoy!

Serves: 6-8

Try topping this zesty meatloaf with guacamole and fresh cilantro. You can also double the recipe and freeze one for a quick and easy weeknight meal, pull from the freezer in the morning and reheat at night.

Lemon Zested Shrimps

Ingredients

½ Tablespoon of coconut oil

½ teaspoon of ground turmeric

12 large shrimps,

¼ cup of olive oil

¼ cup of fresh lemon juice

1 small onion, finely diced

½ Tablespoon of lemon zest

2 cloves of garlic, minced

Half Tablespoon of grated ginger

Directions

1. Peel and devein the shrimps.

2. In a mixing bowl, combine the olive oil, fresh lemon juice, lemon zest, ginger, onion, garlic and ground turmeric. Mix well.

3. Put the shrimps in this mixture. Flip around the shrimps so that they are thoroughly coated in the spice mixture.

4. Cover this bowl with plastic wrap and place it in the refrigerator. Allow it to marinade for at least two hours.

5. When the shrimps are marinated, take them out the refrigerator.

6. Heat the coconut oil in a non-stick pan over medium high flame.

7. Put the shrimps in the pan. Make sure you just put the shrimps and not its marinade.

8. Cook for about ten minutes while stirring frequently, until the shrimps become pink, then add in the marinade.

9. Cook while stirring constantly till the mixture comes to a boil.

10. Take it out in a serving platter and serve immediately!

Chicken Veggie Soup

Ingredients

1 whole chicken, de-boned

2 zucchinis, thinly sliced

3 cloves garlic, minced

1 bay leaf

1 sprig rosemary

5 big, fresh tomatoes, diced

1 yellow onion, finely chopped

2 carrots diced

1 bunch celery, diced

1 tsp. black pepper

1 tsp. all-spice

6 cups water

Directions

1. In a large skillet, combine the chicken, onion, garlic, rosemary, bay leaf, pepper and water and bring to a boil. Let it simmer on low heat for 2 hours. Discard the bay leaf and rosemary and add all the remaining ingredients. Cover and bring to a boil. Cook for about 20 minutes until the vegetables are soft.

2. Enjoy!

Sweet & Sour Pork

Ingredients

1 kg boneless pork loin, cubed

1 ripe pineapple, diced

2 cloves garlic, minced

½ cup orange juice, freshly squeezed

½ tsp. salt

½ tsp. ground cinnamon

1 medium red onion, chopped

¼ cup raisins

½ tsp. cayenne pepper

½ tsp. ground black pepper

¼ cup grated coconut

1 tart apple, peeled and diced

Directions

1. In a slow cooker, mix the orange juice with all the dry ingredients until the mixture starts boiling gently. Add the garlic, apple, raisins, onion and coconut; stirring all the time. Pour in the pork into the slow cooker.

2. Cover and cook on very low heat for about 5 hours. At this point the pork is very tender and you are ready to serve.

3. Enjoy!

Liver Made Colorful

Ingredients

1kg liver, cubed, all fat trimmed off

1 tbsp. olive oil

1 large onion, finely chopped

½ tsp. salt

1 large red pepper, cut into long strips

1 bunch fresh coriander

1 tsp. all-spice

½ tsp. cayenne pepper

½ tsp. black pepper

Directions

1. Heat a wok over medium heat and pour in the olive oil. Add the liver and turn frequently until evenly browned and crispy on the outside. Add the onion and continue mixing until soft.

2. Pour in all the dry ingredients and reduce the heat to the very minimum. Add a little water and cover the wok and let it cook for 20 minutes.

3. Add the pepper stripes together with the coriander and continue turning for one minute and you are ready to serve!

4. Enjoy!

Crispy Duck & Baked Vegetables

Ingredients

2 duck legs, skin on

1 zucchini, chopped

1 rutabaga, chopped

1 cup Brussels sprouts, quartered

1 small yellow onion, chopped

2 cups chicken stock

Coarse sea salt

Freshly ground pepper

Directions

1. Preheat oven to 400 degrees Fahrenheit.

2. Heat a large, cast iron skillet over medium-high heat and add the duck legs, skin side down. Cook for about 10 minutes, until the skin is crispy. Season with salt and pepper and flip. Cook for another minute or two (they will not be cooked through) and remove to a plate.

3. Add the chopped vegetables to the pan and season with salt and pepper. Cook for 10-15 minutes until they begin to brown.

4. Add the duck legs back to the pan, nestling between the vegetables. Add enough chicken stock to the pan to come about half way up the duck legs.

5. Bring to a simmer and place the whole skillet into the oven.

6. Bake 30 minutes, turn heat down to 350 degrees and continue to bake another 30 minutes.

7. Remove from oven, allow to rest for 10 minutes, and divide between two plates.

Roasted Rack of Lamb with Blackberry Sauce

Ingredients

2 racks of lamb, frenched (bones in), about ½ pound each

2 tablespoons grass-fed butter

2 tablespoons ghee

1 tablespoon fresh rosemary, chopped

1 tablespoon fresh thyme

2 cloves of garlic, minced

Coarse sea salt and freshly ground pepper to taste

For the sauce

¼ cup balsamic vinegar

¾ cup blackberries, fresh or frozen

½ cup water

Directions

1. Melt the butter and 1 tablespoon of the ghee together in the microwave and stir in the garlic, rosemary, and thyme.

2. Evenly spread the herb butter onto the lamb and season generously with salt and pepper. Place in a large plastic bag or container and let marinate, in the refrigerator, for at least 1 hour.

3. Preheat the oven to 400 degrees Fahrenheit.

4. In a large skillet, heat 1 tablespoon of ghee over high heat. Once the pan is very hot, sear each rack of lamb, meat side down first for 2-3 minutes. Flip and sear the opposite side for 2 minutes.

5. Place the lamb racks, fat side up in a roasting pan and cook for 7 minutes. Lower heat to 325 degrees and cook for an additional 15 minutes or until a meat thermometer reads 125 degrees. Be careful not to overcook the lamb. *To prevent the bones from burning, wrap in tin foil.

6. Remove from the oven and let rest.

7. To prepare the balsamic blackberry sauce, heat the blackberries and water in a small saucepan over medium heat. Bring to a boil while mashing the blackberries with the back of a wooden spoon. Simmer for 5 minutes.

8. Pour the blackberries through a fine mesh strainer to remove the seeds and return the saucepan.

9. Add the balsamic vinegar and bring to a boil. Let simmer for 10 minutes, or until thickened.

10. To serve; drizzle each rack of lamb with the balsamic blackberry sauce.

Lamb Ragu with Celery Root Pasta

Ingredients:

1 celery root, spiralized

400g lean minced lamb

½ carrot, finely chopped

½ yellow onion, finely chopped

1 clove garlic, minced

½ celery stalk, finely chopped

250 g crushed tomatoes

½ tsp fresh thyme, chopped

½ tsp fresh rosemary, chopped

½ tbsp. olive oil

½ tbsp. tomato paste

¼ tsp red pepper flakes

1tbsp fresh mint, chopped

½ cup homemade chicken broth

1 tsp ground cumin

Kosher salt and freshly ground pepper to taste

Directions:

1. Combine the minced lamb, rosemary, cumin, thyme, garlic, salt and pepper in a pot and place over medium heat. Use a wooden spoon to loosen

the lumps and cook until it is well browned. Stir in the celery, carrot, onion and red pepper flakes and cook for about 5 minutes until the vegetables become soft.

2. Add the tomatoes and stir in the tomato paste and the stock. Once the sauce starts boiling, lower the heat and bring to a gentle simmer for 20 minutes.

3. Meanwhile, add the olive oil in a large skillet and place over medium heat, then sauté the celery root noodles. Cover and cook for up to 10 minutes until the noodles are al dente, stirring occasionally. Add a bit of the broth if the noodles start sticking to the bottom.

4. Divide the cooked noodles into serving bowls together with the lamb ragu and garnish with fresh mint.

5. Enjoy!

Pork Meatloaf with Sun Dried Tomato & Mushrooms

Ingredients

¼ cup mushrooms, dried

900g grass fed minced beef

½ cup sun-dried tomatoes

2 pcs Seitan bacon

1 free range egg

4 cloves garlic, crushed

1 small red onion, diced

¼ cup fresh basil, chopped

½ cup fresh parsley, chopped

1 jalapeno, seeded (optional), minced

1 tsp chili powder

½ tsp freshly ground black pepper

1 tsp coarse sea salt

<u>Top glaze:</u>

¼ cup mushrooms plus 2 tbsp. liquid from mushrooms

¼ cup sun-dried tomatoes, plus 2 tbsp. water from the tomatoes

1 tsp olive oil

1 clove garlic

Directions

1. Place the dried mushrooms in a bowl and cover them with water for 45 minutes, don't pour out the water. Do the same for the dried tomatoes.

2. Now preheat your oven to 375 F.

3. Combine all the meatloaf ingredients until well combined but not over mixed. Scoop the meat mix into your loaf pan and even out the top. Put in the oven and bake for an hour. Meanwhile pulse all the glaze ingredients in your food processor.

4. Once the cook time has elapsed, remove from oven and drain off most of the fat from the meat pan and brush with the pureed glaze. Bake for another 20 minutes until the top caramelizes.

5. Drain off more fat if need be then let sit for 10 minutes before serving. Enjoy!

Caribbean Salad with Monk Fish

Ingredients

1360g monk fish meat, cooked

1 (green and yellow) pepper, seeded and cut into strips

1 medium white onion

8 cups watercress or other leafy greens of choice

4 stalks celery, diced

½ cup extra virgin olive oil

2 lemons, cut into wedges

1 avocado, cut into cubes

Freshly ground black pepper

Directions

1. Place the monk fish meat on a clean surface and chop it up into bite sized pieces. Toss in a large bowl together with the celery, peppers, onion, pepper then drizzle with olive oil.

2. Divide the leafy greens in four salad bowls and add the lobster mix. Arrange the avocado on top and squeeze a lemon wedge over each bowl and garnish with the remaining wedges.

3. Serve immediately. Enjoy!

Chili Bison Stew

Ingredients

1 pound grass-fed bison, ground

2 tablespoons olive oil

1 large sweet potato, cubed

1 medium yellow onion, diced

1 (14 oz.) can fire roasted tomatoes

2 tablespoons tomato paste

2 cloves of garlic, minced

2 tablespoons chili powder

2 teaspoons cumin

2 bay leaves

¼ teaspoon cinnamon

2 teaspoons salt

1 teaspoon pepper

1 ½ cups beef broth

Cilantro and lime wedges to garnish

Directions

1. In a 6 quart Dutch oven, or other large pot, heat the olive oil over medium-high heat and cook the ground bison until browned.

2. Add the onion and garlic and cook until the onion is translucent.

3. Add the cubed sweet potatoes, tomatoes, and tomato paste and cook for 5 minutes.

4. Add all of the seasonings and slowly stir in the beef broth. Bring to a simmer.

5. Cover, reduce heat to low, and cook for 30-45 minutes until the sweet potatoes are tender.

6. Serve with fresh cilantro and a squeeze of lime.

7. Enjoy!

Fried Pork on Turnip Rice

Ingredients:

Pork:

450g pork shoulder

2 cloves garlic, minced

1 tsp tomato paste

1 tsp hoisin sauce

½ tbsp. coconut aminos

½ tsp sweet paprika

¼ tsp sesame oil

½ tbsp. sherry

¼ tsp five spice powder

½ tbsp. raw honey

½ tbsp. extra virgin olive oil

½ tbsp. hot water

A good pinch salt and white pepper

Turnip rice:

3 turnips

1 white onion

2 eggs

1 tbsp. coconut aminos

1 tsp sesame oil

½ tbsp. extra virgin olive oil

4 scallions

Directions

1. Whisk together all the ingredients of the pork marinade in a mixing bowl and set aside 2 tablespoons. Cut the pork into about 3" pieces and place in a zip lock bag or airtight container, then pour in the marinade. Shake well and chill in the fridge for at least 4 hours or preferably overnight.

2. Meanwhile, chop the scallions and the white onion and place in the fridge.

3. Once the pork is ready, pre-heat the oven to 455F and line your baking tray with kitchen foil, then place a rack on top.

4. Place the marinated pork on the rack for about 25 minutes and baste it using the juices that have poured on the baking tray plus the remaining marinade. Bake for 20 more minutes, then broil the pork for 2 minutes to make it crisp on the outside but don't let it burn.

5. Remove the pork from the oven and brush it with the reserved 2 tablespoons of marinade and let it stand for 10 minutes before cutting it up.

6. Now peel the turnips and spiralize into noodles. Place the noodles in a food processor and pulse until it forms turnip rice then set aside.

7. Place a medium skillet on medium heat, coat with cooking spray then scramble the eggs and transfer them to a plate.

8. Wipe the skillet and pour in the olive oil and place on medium heat. Sauté the onions for 3 minutes then stir in the pork and turnip rice. Allow to cook for 5 minutes till the turnip becomes soft. Stir in the sesame oil, coconut aminos, scrambled eggs, scallions and white pepper and cook for 2 minutes until they are heated through.

9. Enjoy!

Island Salmon with Mange Chili Salsa

Ingredients

Salmon:

4 salmon fillets with the skin on, about 6oz each

Freshly ground pepper

Flaky Maldon sea salt

Coconut oil

Salsa:

1 large mango, peeled and cubed

2 tsp fresh coriander, finely chopped

¾ tsp Serrano chili, seeded and minced

½ red bell pepper, diced

½ red onion, finely chopped

2 tbsp. freshly squeezed lime juice

Sea salt

Directions

1. Start by preheating your oven to 350 F and set your baking rack at the center position.

2. Gently rub the fillets with salt and pepper and set aside.

3. Place an oven proof pan over medium heat and add about 2 tablespoons of coconut oil. Once the oil is shimmering hot, gently place the salmon on the pan with the skin side up and cook for 3 minutes then flip over and cook for a minute. Turn off the heat and place the pan in the oven and bake for 10 minutes until cooked through.

4. Meanwhile, combine all the salsa ingredients and chill in the fridge.

5. Once the salmon is ready, serve with the salsa and enjoy!

Tip: the salsa tastes even better when you prepare it at least 6 hours in advance so the flavors have time to meld.

Broiled Lemon & Garlic Mackerel

Ingredients

4 mackerel fillets

sea salt and ground black pepper to taste

3 cloves garlic (finely chopped)

1/2 tsp sweet paprika powder

4 Tbsp olive oil

12 slices lemon

Coconut oil

Directions

1. First, preheat the oven's broiler and grease a baking dish with coconut oil.

2. Generously rub each mackerel fillet (from both sides) with olive oil. Put the fish with the skin side down into the prepared baking dish.

3. Season each fillet with salt and pepper to taste and sweet paprika. Add evenly garlic over the fish. Cut the lemon in slices and top each fillet with two lemon slices.

4. Bake the fillets under the broiler 6 - 7 minutes.

5. Serve hot with your favorite vegetables.

Pumpkin & Sun-dried Tomato Pork Stew

Ingredients

2,5 lb boneless pork

3 cups cubed pumpkin

1/4 cup sundried tomatoes

4 garlic cloves, minced

1 Tbsp coriander

3 Tbsp smoked paprika

4 dried red chiles, chopped

1 Tbsp of oregano

1 Tbsp black pepper (fresh ground)

1 tsp cinnamon

3 Tbsp coconut oil

1/4 cup sundried tomatoes

2 onion (chopped)

salt and pepper to taste

cilantro and parsley for garnish

8-10 cups water

Directions

1. First, cut the pork into small cubes.

2. In a small bowl combine all the spices and rub the mixture onto the pork. Add a cooking fat in a large pot. Add the pork and cook about 7-8 minutes. Remove pork from the pan and set aside.

3. Add the chilles, sundried tomatoes, garlic and onions. Cook for about 3 minutes more.

4. Return the pork to the pan and add about 8-10 cups of water. Bring to a boil, reduce heat and cook covered for about 3 hours.

5. When ready, add the pumpkin cubes and cook for another 30 minutes.

6. Garnish with your cilantro and parsley and serve hot.

Chicken Stuffed Peppers

Ingredients

4 bell peppers (any color)

1 pound ground chicken

½ head cauliflower

1 yellow onion, diced

2 carrots, peeled and diced

4 cloves of garlic, minced

1 (6 ounce) can tomato paste

3 tablespoons Italian seasoning

¼ cup beef stock

Sea salt and pepper to taste

Directions

1. Preheat oven to 350 degrees Fahrenheit. Place the cauliflower, onion, carrots, and garlic in a food processor. Pulse until finely ground.

2. Cut the tops off of your peppers and remove the seeds.

3. Mix the vegetables with the ground chicken, and tomato paste. Season with Italian seasoning and salt and pepper.

4. Spoon the mixture into the peppers and place in baking dish. Make sure to place the pepper tops back on.

5. Pour the beef stock in the bottom of the dish and cook for 45-60 minutes, until the peppers are tender and the chicken is cooked through.

6. Enjoy!

Serves: 4

Bell peppers have quite a bit going for them. They're low in calories, high in fiber, and an excellent source of vitamins A and C.

Slow Cooker Chicken Chili Verde

Ingredients

2 pounds boneless chicken breasts and/or thighs

2 jalapeno peppers, deseeded and cut in half

2 poblano peppers, deseeded and cut in half

8-10 tomatillos, husked and cut in half

2 tablespoons olive oil

1 small onion, diced

2 cloves of garlic, minced

½ cup lime juice

2 teaspoons oregano

1 teaspoon cumin

sea salt and pepper to taste

2 cups chicken broth or water

Directions

1. Preheat oven to 450 degrees Fahrenheit.

2. Place the jalapenos, poblanos, and tomatillos on a metal baking sheet and drizzle with the olive oil. Cook for 20-30 minutes, until charred on the outside. Allow to cool and run the peppers under cool water to remove the charred skin.

3. In a food processor or blender, pulse the cooked peppers and tomatillos with the onion, garlic, and lime juice until well combined.

4. Place the chicken in your slow cooker, cover with the pepper/tomatillo puree, and sprinkle with spices.

5. Pour the broth over everything and cook on low for 8 hours.

6. Garnish with lime wedges and cilantro, if desired.

Serves: 5-6

Tomatillos look like a small green tomato, but they're actually related to berries. They contain significant amounts of fiber, very few calories, and are low in fat.

Cilantro Lime Halibut

Ingredients

4 halibut filets

Juice of 2 limes

1 cup cilantro

½ cup olive oil + 3 tablespoons

Sea salt and pepper m

Directions

1. Blend the lime juice, cilantro, ½ cup olive oil, and salt and pepper in a blender or food processor until well combined.

2. Place the halibut in a large Ziploc bag and pour the mixture into it. Toss to coat well.

3. Refrigerate for 10-15 minutes.

4. Heat the 3 tablespoons olive oil in a large skillet over medium high heat.

5. Add the halibut and cook for about 4-5 minutes per side.

6. Serve alongside salad greens or vegetable of your choice.

Serves: 4

Halibut is among one of the best sources of omega-3 fatty acids. It has a firm texture and mild taste. If unavailable in your area, try substituting with mahi-mahi or red snapper.

Beef and Broccoli Stir Fry

Serves: 4

Serving Size: About 1 cup

Ingredients

Marinade:

1 shallot, minced

2 cloves garlic, minced

½ cup water

½ cup orange juice

1/3 cup coconut aminos

1/3 cup coconut oil

4 green onion, sliced

1" piece of ginger, grated

1 teaspoon vinegar

Salt and pepper to taste

1 pound grass-fed beef, cut into ½" pieces

2 cups broccoli florets

1 (8 ounce package) mushrooms, thinly sliced

3 carrots, thinly sliced

1 yellow onion, thinly sliced

2 tablespoons coconut oil

Directions

1. Whisk the marinade ingredients together in a small bowl until well combined. Place the beef in a separate bowl and cover with half the marinade.

2. Heat the coconut oil in a skillet over medium heat. Cook the mushrooms until lightly browned. Add the sliced onion, carrots, and broccoli and cook until tender.

3. Remove from skillet and set aside.

4. Add the beef to the skillet and cook about 8-10 minutes.

5. Return the mushrooms, onion, and broccoli to the pan and stir in the remainder of the marinade.

6. Cook and stir until simmering and heated through.

7. Serve and enjoy!

When selecting beef for a stir fry, choose a cut that is tender and will benefit from the quick cooking method. A sirloin cut is a great choice, while a flank steak or bottom round may need a little bit longer in the marinade to tenderize.

Chicken and Sweet Potato Pot Pies

Ingredients

2 boneless, skinless chicken breasts

2 small sweet potatoes

Coarse sea salt and black pepper

Juice of one orange

6 cups baby spinach

½ cup toasted almonds, chopped

¼ cup coconut milk (canned)

Directions

1. Preheat oven to 350 degrees Fahrenheit.

2. Season the chicken breasts with salt and pepper. Place the sweet potatoes in a large baking dish along with the chicken breasts.

3. Pour the orange juice over the chicken and cover the pan with foil. Bake for 30-35 minutes until the sweet potatoes are fork tender. Set aside to cool slightly.

4. In a medium pan, sauté the spinach until just wilted.

5. Chop the cooked chicken and add to a large bowl. Using a spoon, scoop out the flesh of the sweet potatoes. Add in the spinach, toasted almonds, and coconut milk. Gently fold until well combined.

6. Divide the mixture between 2 oven safe crocks or large ramekins.

7. Place under the broiler for 1-2 minutes until golden brown on top.

8. Serve and enjoy!

Serves: 1

Sweet potatoes are a great source of vitamin A, which supports the immune system. Just one serving contains more than 100% of the daily recommended amount of vitamin A.

Vegetable Beef Soup

Inbredients

¼ cup butter

1 pound ground beef

1 yellow onion, chopped

3 carrots, peeled and chopped

3 celery ribs, chopped

4 cloves of garlic, minced

2 tablespoons tomato paste

1 (15 ounce can) diced tomatoes

8 cups beef broth (homemade, if available)

3 cups baby spinach or kale

Sea salt and freshly ground pepper

Directions

1. In a large stock pot, sauté the onion, carrot, and celery in the butter. Cook until the onions are translucent. Add the garlic and season with salt and pepper.

2. While the vegetables are cooking, brown the ground beef in a separate pan.

3. Stir the tomato paste into the vegetables, add the cooked ground beef and beef bone broth and bring to a boil.

4. Reduce heat to low and let simmer for about 15 minutes.

5. Add the spinach and cook a few more minutes, until the spinach is wilted. Season with salt and pepper to taste.

6. Serve and enjoy!

Serves: 6-8

Try doubling this recipe and freezing leftovers in individual serving sizes. It packs up great for work or school.

Blackened Tuna with Mango Salsa

Ingredients

1 ½ to 2 pounds of wild caught tuna filets

3 tablespoons coconut oil, melted

2 teaspoons paprika

1 teaspoon garlic powder

1 teaspoon onion powder

½ teaspoon thyme

½ teaspoon black pepper

½ teaspoon cayenne pepper

½ teaspoon dried basil

½ teaspoon dried oregano

Mango Salsa:

1 large, ripe mango, diced

1 avocado, diced

8-10 cherry tomatoes, quartered

½ red onion, diced

¼ cup cilantro, chopped

1 jalapeno, seeded and diced

Juice of ½ a lime

½ teaspoon salt

Directions

1. Combine the salsa ingredients in a bowl and mix well. Refrigerate until ready to serve.

2. Preheat a grill pan or cast iron skillet over medium-high heat. Combine all of the spices in a small bowl. Mix well.

3. Coat the tuna filets with the melted coconut oil and rub with the spice mixture.

4. Place the tuna filets in the pan and cook for about 2-3 minutes. Carefully flip the tuna, and cook for about 2-3 minutes or until it's reached your desired level of doneness.

5. To serve, place on a bed of greens and spoon the mango salsa on top. Enjoy!

Serves: 4

Wild caught tuna is high in selenium, an essential trace mineral that is important for cognitive function and a healthy immune system.

Slow Cooker Balsamic Roast Beef

Ingredients

3-4 pound chuck roast

1 yellow onion, diced

6 cloves garlic, minced

1 cup beef stock

½ balsamic vinegar

2 tablespoons coconut aminos

Pinch of red pepper flakes

Sea salt and pepper to taste

Directions

1. Place the roast in your slow cooker fat side down.

2. Add the remaining ingredients over the top of the roast.

3. Cover and cook on low for 6-8 hours. It should shred easily with a fork when it's done.

4. Remove the roast from the slow cooker and blend the juices, onion, and garlic with an immersion blender.

5. Serve the gravy alongside the roast beef and your favorite vegetable.

6. Enjoy!

Serves: 5-6

Red meat is an important part of keeping your iron levels up. Iron deficiency can lead to anemia, headaches, and most commonly, low energy.

Shredded Chicken with Roasted Peppers

Ingredients

1 pound boneless, skinless chicken breasts

½ cup chicken broth

3 bell peppers (any color), diced

1 red onion, diced

1 jalapeno, deseeded and diced

2 cloves of garlic, minced

2 cups salsa

1 teaspoon cumin

2 teaspoons chili powder

Sea salt and pepper to taste

1 avocado, diced

Directions

1. Place chicken breasts and broth in the bottom of your slow cooker.

2. Sprinkle with the cumin, chili powder, and salt and pepper.

3. Add the salsa and diced onion. Cook on low for 6-8 hours.

4. Once the chicken is done cooking, shred with tongs or two forks.

5. Sauté the bell peppers and jalapeno over medium-high heat, until well roasted.

6. Add the peppers to the slow cooker and stir to mix well.

7. Cook for an additional 20 minutes.

8. Top with avocado before serving.

Serves: 4

This recipe can easily be done on the stovetop instead of a slow cooker. Just use a heavy bottomed stock pot and cook on low for 2-3 hours.

Turkey and Butternut Squash Chili

Ingredients

2 pounds ground turkey

2 tablespoons olive oil

1 teaspoon smoked paprika

1 teaspoon sea salt

½ teaspoon chipotle powder

1 yellow onion, diced

1 large butternut squash, peeled and diced

1 (14 ounce can) diced tomatoes

2 tablespoons tomato paste

Sea salt and black pepper to taste

Sliced green onions (garnish)

Fresh cilantro (optional)

Directions

1. Heat olive in a large stock pot over medium-high heat.

2. Add the ground turkey and season with smoked paprika, salt, and chipotle powder. Cook until browned.

3. Stir in the onion and butternut squash. Mix well.

4. Add the tomatoes, tomato paste, and beef broth. Season with salt and pepper.

5. Reduce heat to medium, cover, and cook for 45 minutes to an hour, stirring every so often.

6. The chili is ready once the butternut squash is tender.

7. Top with sliced green onion and fresh cilantro. Serve!

Serves: 6-8

Beans are excluded from this whole foods diet because they aren't a dense protein source and contain 2-3 times the amount of carbohydrates than protein. They also contain high amounts of phytates which bind to minerals, rendering them unavailable to our bodies.

Spicy potatoes with roasted cod

Ingredients

12 small red potatoes, sliced

4 halibut fillets, skinned

2 tbsp. extra virgin olive oil

2 bunches scallions, ends trimmed

½ tsp chili powder

1 lemon, zested

Directions

1. Set your oven to 425F.
2. Toss the sliced potatoes with salt, pepper, chili powder and 1 tablespoon of olive oil on a rimmed baking sheet.
3. Roast for 25 minutes until soft and golden brown. Toss the potato slices once to allow for even cooking.
4. Place the fillets and scallions in another baking sheet and season well with salt and pepper. Drizzle the remaining olive oil over the fish and sprinkle with lemon zest.
5. After 10 minutes of cook time for the potatoes, place the fish in the oven and bake for 15 minutes until the halibut turns opaque on all sides.
6. Serve the potato slices, halibut and scallions. Cut the lemon in half and squeeze over your plate.
7. Enjoy!

Tasty stuffed steak roulades

Ingredients

225g flank steak

2 cups fresh spinach with stems removed

¼ cup olive tapenade

1 tsp Dijon mustard

6 cups mixed greens

1 tbsp. red wine vinegar

2 tbsp. olive oil

Freshly ground black pepper to taste

Kosher salt to taste

Directions

1. Set your grill to medium high. Next, cut the steak horizontally but not all the way through. It should resemble an open book.
2. Spread the olive tapenade followed by the spinach. Roll up the steak and use kitchen twine to secure it.
3. Season the outer part with salt and pepper and grill for about 15 minutes, covered. Let stand for 5-10 minutes before slicing it up.
4. As the steak is cooking, whisk the olive oil, mustard, vinegar, salt and pepper. Toss in the mixed greens and serve with the stuffed steak.
5. Enjoy!

Slow Cooker Chicken and Sweet Potato Stew

INGREDIENTS

1 pound boneless, skinless chicken breasts

1 yellow onion, diced

3 carrots, peeled and diced

1 large sweet potato, peeled and diced

4 cloves of garlic, minced

2 cups homemade chicken broth

1 can tomato paste

3 tablespoons balsamic vinegar

2 teaspoons whole grain mustard

2 bay leaves

2 cups baby spinach

Sea salt and pepper to taste

Directions

1. Cut chicken breasts into chunks and add to the pot of your slow cooker.

2. Add the onion, carrots, sweet potato, garlic, chicken broth, tomato paste, balsamic vinegar, mustard, and bay leaves. Stir to combine. Season with salt and pepper.

3. Place slow cooker on high for 4-5 hours or low for 6-8 hours.

4. An hour before serving, add the spinach and mix well.

5. Serve and enjoy! Store any leftovers in an airtight container in the refrigerator or freezer.

Serves: 4-6

The joy of slow cookers! Just dump everything in first thing in the morning and dinner is taken care of! This hearty stew makes a satisfying meal on a cold night.

Thai Stir Fry

INGREDIENTS

Marinade:

1 shallot, minced

2 cloves garlic, minced

½ cup water

½ cup orange juice

1/3 cup coconut aminos

1/3 cup coconut oil

4 green onion, sliced

1" piece of ginger, grated

1 teaspoon vinegar

Salt and pepper to taste

1 pound boneless, skinless chicken breasts, cubed

½ cup broccoli florets

1 (8 ounce package) mushrooms, sliced

2 carrots, shredded

2 zucchini, spiralized (or made into ribbons with a vegetable peeler)

½ yellow onion, sliced

2 tablespoons coconut oil

Directions

1. Whisk the marinade ingredients together in a small bowl until well combined. Place the chicken in a separate bowl and cover with half the marinade.

2. Heat the coconut oil in a skillet over medium heat. Cook the mushrooms until lightly browned. Add the sliced onion and broccoli and cook until tender.

3. Remove from skillet and set aside.

4. Add the chicken to the skillet and cook about 10-15 minutes. Toss in the zucchini noodles and shredded carrots. Cook until the zucchini noodles are tender, about 2-3 minutes.

5. Return the mushrooms, onion, and broccoli to the pan and stir in the remainder of the marinade.

6. Cook and stir until simmering and heated through.

7. Serve and enjoy!

Serves: 4

If you don't have a spiralizer for the zucchini, you can use a vegetable peeler to make long ribbons, or just chop the zucchini into half-moon shapes. You can also swap the zucchini for yellow squash or spaghetti squash.

Braised chicken with spring veggies

Ingredients

6 chicken thighs (bone-in)

4 carrots, cut into sticks

2 tbsp. freshly chopped chives

1 small bunch celery, cut into sticks

1 tbsp. olive oil

12 radishes, cut in half

1 cup low-sodium chicken broth

Freshly ground black pepper to taste

Kosher salt to taste

Directions

1. Pour the oil in a large Dutch oven over medium heat. Season the chicken with salt and pepper and add them to the Dutch oven for browning. Cook for 7 minutes or until evenly browned then set aside.
2. Discard the excess fat from the Dutch oven and stir in the broth. Add the veggies then top with the browned chicken and cook for about 20 minutes over medium-low heat.
3. Sprinkle with the chives and you are ready to indulge.
4. Enjoy!

Dessert Recipes

Slim-down vanilla flavored mocha Frappuccino

Ingredients

2 cups unsweetened strong coffee, frozen

1 tsp pure vanilla extract

½ cup almond milk, unsweetened

2 packets stevia (natural sweetener with zero calories)

1 tsp pre cocoa powder, unsweetened

A small pinch of sea salt

Directions

1. Mix instant coffee and water, in desired proportions and stir well until the coffee dissolves. Pour this in a shallow dish, cover and place in your freezer for a minimum of 4 hours or better yet, overnight.
2. Once the coffee has set, combine it with the remaining ingredients in a power blender ad pulse until perfectly combined.
3. Serve in a glass. You can add some berries for a negative calorie antioxidant punch.
4. Enjoy!

Skinny green tea-berry freeze

Ingredients

2 cups strong-brewed green tea

4 large strawberries

2 packets stevia (zero calorie natural sweetener)

½ cup crushed ice or 5 ice cubes

Lemon wedges for serving

Directions

1. Combine all the ingredients in your blender and pulse until evenly combined.
2. Serve in 2 tall glasses and garnish with lemon wedges.
3. Enjoy!

5-minute super moist chocolate cake

Ingredients

1 box Betty Crocker Dark chocolate (Super moist Cake Mix)

3 free range eggs

1 extra ripe banana

1 1/3 cups water

Non-stick olive oil cooking spray

Directions

1. Mash up the banana in a big bowl and whisk it together with the eggs and water until smooth.
2. Add in the cake mix and stir vigorously until smooth.
3. Lightly spray ramekins with cooking spray and spoon the batter into them until 2/3 full.
4. Microwave 2 ramekins at a time on medium to high temperature setting and microwave for 5 minutes.
5. Use a toothpick to check if your cakes are done. If the cake sticks, then give it 30 seconds until the cake crumbles on the toothpick.
6. Top with pure pomegranate juice for increased antioxidant power.
7. Enjoy!

Yummy apple chips

Ingredients

2 granny smith apples

1 tsp stevia (zero calorie natural sweetener)

1 tsp ground cinnamon

A touch of canola cooking spray

Directions

1. Use a mandolin or a very sharp knife to thinly slice the apples, crosswise. Layer the apple slices on a baking sheet and lightly spray with canola cooking spray. Top with cinnamon and stevia and bake at the bottom part of the oven at 350F until the chips are nice and crisp for about 2 hours.
2. Enjoy!

Tasty crust-less apple pie

Ingredients

1 large green apple

2 packets stevia (zero calorie natural sweetener)

½ tsp ground cinnamon

Directions

1. Peel your apple then slice it thinly then cut the slices in quarters.
2. Combine the apple, stevia and cinnamon in a non-stick pan and cook on medium – high until soft but with a bite to it, or if you prefer, until mushy.
3. Enjoy!

Barbequed Peaches & Plum with Cream Cheese

Ingredients:

10 ripe peaches, cut in halves and pitted

24 purple/ red plums cut in halves and pitted, with 4 sliced thinly

2 tbsp. freshly squeezed lemon juice

1 cup water

½ cup raw honey

6 tbsp. organic butter, melted

Cream cheese for serving

Directions:

1. Prepare your grill and set to medium heat.
2. Meanwhile, place a medium saucepan over medium to high heat and add the water, sliced plums and ¾ cup of honey. Once it starts boiling, cover and bring to a gentle simmer for 10 minutes. The plums should be super soft. Place the cooked plums in your food processor and pulse until it forms a smooth puree. Scoop the puree into a small bowl and combine with lemon juice.

3. Now, whisk the melted butter with the remaining honey and set aside. Grill the peaches and plums over medium heat until desired tenderness is achieved, that's about 6 minutes. Baste the fruits with the butter-honey paste and turn them once on the grill. Keep grilling until they caramelize and char slightly say about 2 more minutes.

4. Serve the grilled fruits on fruit bowls and drizzle with the plum puree. Top with a generous dollop of cream cheese and enjoy!

Grilled Pineapple Sundaes with Shredded Coconut

Ingredients:

1 whole ripe pineapple. Peeled, cored and cut in rings

½ cup shredded coconut, sweetened

2 tsp vegetable oil

Frozen vanilla yogurt, fat free

Mint sprigs

Directions:

1. Prepare a grill and set to medium. Lightly brush the pineapple rings with vegetable oil and place on the grill. Turn the pineapples once or twice and grill until they are soft and a bit charred, for about 8 minutes. Transfer the pineapples to a cutting board and chop them up.
2. Now toast the shredded coconut in a small pan over low heat and serve on a plate.
3. Serve the fro-yo (frozen yogurt) into sundae glasses or ice cream bowl and place the grilled pineapple on top, sprinkle with toasted coconut and garnish with mint sprigs. Serve immediately.

Grilled Pound Cake topped with Mixed Berries

Ingredients:

4 (1/2") paleo pound cake slices

450g mixed berries (strawberries and blueberries)

¾ tsp arrowroot powder

1 tbsp. freshly squeezed lemon juice

1 tsp lemon zest, finely grated

2 tbsp. organic unsalted butter

1/8 cup raw honey

4 (12") heavy aluminum foil squares

Strawberry ice cream(see recipe in snack section) or crème fraiche for serving

Directions:

1. Prepare your grill and set to medium heat.
2. Toss the berries with honey, lemon juice and zest and arrowroot powder in a medium bowl.
3. Now, spread out the aluminum foil squares and place a ¼ tablespoon of butter at the center of each sheet. Top with the fruit mixture and fold two sides of the sheet followed by the other two sides. Ensure the packs are tightly sealed.
4. Place the packs of the heated grill and grill for 10 minutes until the fruit starts sizzling.

BBQ Berry Crostini with Crème Fraiche

Ingredients:

4 cups fresh mixed berries

3-4 slices original country bread, cut in half cross-wise

1/8 cup pure maple syrup

1 tbsp. natural honey

Organic unsalted butter, softened for brushing

½ cup paleo crème fraiche

A good pinch kosher salt

Directions:

1. Start by lighting an outdoor charcoal fire grill.
2. Combine honey with crème fraiche in a small bowl and whisk thoroughly until they are well blended.
3. Butter both sides of the bread slices and spread with a bit of maple syrup. Grill the bread over medium heat until it is caramelized and crisp for about 3 minutes. Remove from grill and place on a plate to cool off.
4. Place the berries in a mixing bowl and toss with kosher salt and maple syrup. Line the berries on a grill basket or if you don't have one, on a perforated grill pan/ sheet and then grill over medium heat, tossing frequently until they start bursting, that should be about 4-5 minutes. Remove from grill and transfer to a bowl.
5. Top the crostini with warm berries and with generous dollops of honeyed crème fraiche.
6. Enjoy!

Sugar &Dairy Free Brownies

Ingredients

1 tbsp. cocoa powder, unsweetened

1 cup unsweetened coconut

3 dates, seeds removed

Tbsp. extra virgin olive oil

Directions

1. Combine all the ingredients in a food processor and pulse until smooth.
2. Scoop into a small bowl and chill for 10-15 minutes.
3. Slice up and indulge.
4. Enjoy!

Chapter 5:

The Negative Calorie Diet Lifestyle Changes

You are certainly feeling motivated to eat healthy negative calorie foods to help you achieve your ideal body and to exercise more and you are now ready to make positive lifestyle changes that you are going to stick to from now henceforth.

You've probably tried to do this before but it didn't work out for you as you had hoped for. However, this time things are different. For one, you don't have to worry about getting ravenously hungry from a restricted diet. The Negative Calorie Diet is the most indulgent diet on the planet and so making your goals this time will be easier.

However, it is important to note that lifestyle changes are a process that take a lot of time getting used to and you therefore require support.

The fact that you are now ready to make a change is a huge step; the difficult part usually comes in committing and following through with your goals.

Here are a few tips that can set you on the right path of success.

Make a plan that you can follow through

Look at your plan as a road map that is supposed to guide you on this amazing journey of change. Don't stress too much about it. In fact, look at it like an adventure that is going to impact positively on your life.

Be specific with every plan you make and most of all, be realistic. If your plan is to lose weight; how much weight do you want to lose and within what time period?

Small but sure

The best way to meet your goals is to start small by setting daily goals then let these transform into weekly goals. For example you can choose to replace your desserts with a healthy negative calorie food for starters.

Drop one bad habit at a time, don't go cold turkey!

We acquire bad habits over the course of time and so does replacing them with healthy habits this is the surest way to success. Take it one habit after another until finally you start leading a pure negative calorie way of life.

Exercise reigns!

Earlier on we saw that exercise is one of the best metabolism boosters. You also want to tone up your body after losing all that weight and what better way than using exercise to get some beautiful muscles?

The important thing is to choose a workout that works best for you. If you are a no pain no gain' kind of person, then weight lifting might just be the thing for you. If you love adventure, hiking, outdoor running, rock climbing and other outdoor exercises will work perfectly for you. If you love dancing, you can join Zumba classes and so on. Make sure you get a workout that you will be looking forward to going to and not one that you will be looking for excuses not to go to.

Most importantly...

Your body is a temple that deserves to be well taken care of and nourished. Make your health your priority and you will always make the right choices for your body.

The Negative Calorie Diet is the epitome of how you should feed your body. Don't be too hard on yourself either if you slip. Just pick yourself up and resume from where you left of. With time you will find that you will no longer crave junk and over-processed food.

Your body will be so in tune with the Negative Calorie Diet you will only want to eat what you are sure is providing positive nutrition to your body.

In the Negative Calorie Diet, we have nothing like cheating as all our foods are super tasty and super nutritious. The only thing you need to do is to commit to this diet to allow your taste buds to adjust so you can start craving healthy apple chips instead of the fat laden potato chips in food stores.

It's time to make the big negative calorie change!

<u>Conclusion</u>

Thank you again for purchasing The Negative Calorie Diet!

I hope that this guide was able to show you that eating a
healthy diet and leading a healthy lifestyle is as easy as
eating fresh, natural and wholesome foods. This is all you
need to finally lose all the weight that has been bugging
you for the longest of time.

The next step is to 'spring clean' your kitchen and eliminate
all processed foods and replace them with healthy negative
caloric foods that we have looked at in the book. Most
importantly, commit to all the principles we have
addressed in the book for the Negative Calorie Diet to work
for you.

Of all the basic tenets of our lies, health and food are
perhaps the most important. Give the Negative Calorie Diet
an honest try and your life will change forever!

Finally, if you feel that you have received any value from
this book, then I'd like to ask if you would be kind enough
to click on the link below and leave a review on Amazon to
share your positive experience with other readers.
It'd be greatly appreciated!

Made in United States
Orlando, FL
19 October 2022